EATING FOR A's

EATING FOR A's

A month-by-month nutrition and lifestyle guide
to help raise smarter kids
Kindergarten to 6th grade

Second Edition

Kathleen M. Dunn, MPH, RD
Lorna A. Williams, MPH, RD

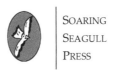

SOARING
SEAGULL
PRESS

Eating for A's
A month-by-month nutrition and lifestyle guide to help raise smarter kids
Second edition

Published by
Soaring Seagull Press
Santa Rosa, CA
www.EatingFor.com

All trademarks and photographs are the property of their respective owners. Photograph on page 10 courtesy of Oakland Athletics; pages 18, 98, 228 and 296 by Cathy Yeulet / Bigstock.com; pages 38, 152 and 240 by Lorna Williams / Soaring Seagull Press; page 58 by Andres Rodriguez / Bigstock.com; pages 86 and 306 by Thomas Perkins / Bigstock.com; page 114 by Wavebreak Media Ltd / Bigstock.com; page 134 by Christophe Rolland / Bigstock.com; page 174 by Eli Mordechai / Bigstock.com; page 184 by Vanessa Bumbeers / Unsplash.com; page 202 by Valeriy Lebedev / Bigstock.com; page 272 by Mandy Godbehear / Bigstock.com; page 316 by Daniel Hurst / Bigstock.com; and back cover by Katharine Noble.

Illustrations | Lorna Williams, Anika Williams
Cover | Lorna Williams, Andy Paolella

Library of Congress Control Number: 2023903460
ISBN: 978-0-9848540-3-5
Printed in the United States of America

Dedication

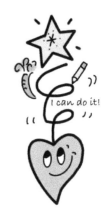

To my husband Chris for his unwavering belief in this project and to the memory of my parents who taught me that achieving life's goals requires the right blend of good nutrition, hard work and confidence—all nourished by a kind heart.

– Kathleen Dunn, MPH, RD

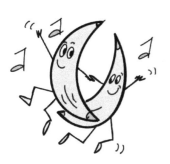

To my husband Brad for his endless support and encouragement, to my children Andrew and Anika who fill my world with joy and laughter and to my parents who lovingly taught me the secret of a life in balance—work hard (thanks, Dad), but remember to take time to dance (thanks, Mom).

– Lorna Williams, MPH, RD

Table of Contents

Part 1

Introduction

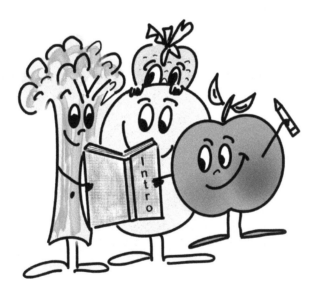

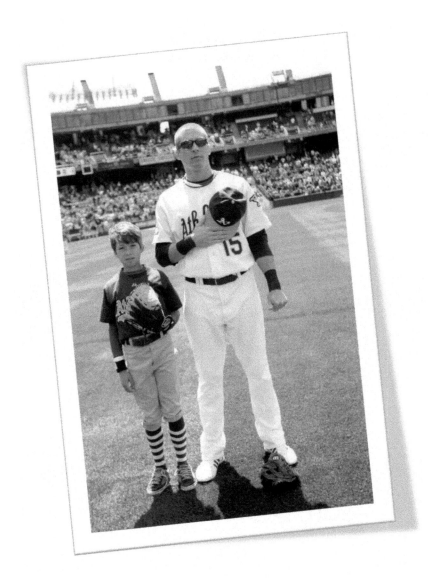

What we think, we become.
— *Buddha*

Chapter 1

Start Here

As registered dietitians, we've heard the collective battle cry from busy parents who want the best for their children: "Give us nutrition tips to help our kids excel in school. No information overload. No complex strategy to learn. Just the need-to-know basics that work with today's hectic lifestyle." If this sounds all too familiar, then this book is for you.

We listened and went to work distilling essential nutrition information into 12 goals that are sure to help your child build the healthy habits that an active mind and optimal learning demand.

Why 12 goals? For most parents of young children, it's second nature to juggle schedules around the months of a typical school year. September typically ushers in the excitement of a new school year, January marks the halfway point and June signals the beginning of long summer days. So, why not apply this same by-the-month mindset to shape healthy, brain-building habits for your kids? After all, behavioral scientists have found that it takes about 28 days to transform a new behavior into a regular habit. What's more, organizing each monthly goal around the activities of a typical school year lets you put them into practice in real life—your real life.

Work Smart, Not Hard

To get the most out of this book, we recommend that you concentrate on one chapter per month. This allows you plenty of time to put each chapter's goal into practice.

With each new chapter, you'll tackle a new goal, but you'll also continue practicing your new habits from previous chapters. With each month, you'll be one step closer to a solid foundation of 12 brain-boosting habits that will help your kids reach their full potential.

To coincide with the school year, start at the chapter that corresponds with the month during which you're reading. For example, if you start reading this book in September, begin with **Chapter 2: September – Family Meals**. If, however, you should open this book in the middle of the school year, say in January, we recommend you start at **Chapter 6: January – Pack a Power Lunch**. In other words, there is no "best" time to start—unless it's now.

A word of caution: Don't be tempted to move ahead. Stay focused on tackling one chapter—and one goal—per month. If you're anxious to do more, explore the extra credit in each chapter. Remember, this is not a race against time. It's a day-to-day approach, and the best way to win is with a slow and steady pace.

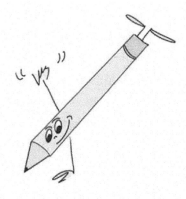

Tips from Parents

As you read, you'll notice each chapter includes "Parent Pearls." These are creative solutions we've learned from parents like you who are eager to encourage better food choices for the entire family, but especially for their young children.

Tips from Experts

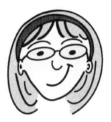

Each chapter also includes information on the latest scientific evidence from experts in the field of nutrition as it relates to each chapter's topic. You'll find these tidbits highlighted in the "Did You Know?" boxes throughout the book.

Setting Goals like a Pro

The best way to establish healthy habits is to set goals. Goals help us achieve what we want; they reflect our purpose and have a wide impact on our lives. In this way, goals are the stepping stones to realizing our dreams. In other words, goals give our lives meaning.

Yet, all too often, people set lofty goals that all but defy the basic laws of physiology. Sadly, these goals are doomed to fail. "We're going to add five more servings of fruit to our daily menu." "We're going to double our fiber intake starting tomorrow." "We're going to eliminate all sugar starting tomorrow." As soon as we hear these grand proclamations from parents who are eager to improve their family's nutrition and lifestyle habits, we have a pretty good idea of the disappointment that lies ahead.

A better approach is to set reasonable goals that you're likely to achieve. Talk with your child and get their input. Encourage them to get a little out of their comfort zone. After all, it's only when we stretch the canvas of life that we can really reach our full potential.

Here's how you can set goals like the pros do. Every effective goal includes five key elements. Goals must be **S**pecific, **M**easurable, **A**ttainable, **R**ealistic and **T**imed. Behavior experts often refer to this type of goal by its acronym, a SMART goal. Read on for a quick primer on how to make sure your goals are SMART goals.

Five Elements of a SMART Goal

1 **A SMART goal is specific.** Let's say your child is on the heavier side, and the excess weight is a concern. For overweight kids, who are otherwise healthy, it's generally recommended to allow them to "grow" into their weight rather than put them on a weight loss diet, so a specific weight loss goal is generally not recommended. Rather, encourage your child to focus on the specific behaviors involved in achieving a

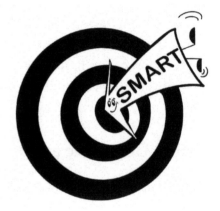

healthy body weight and set goals related to those behaviors. For example, "I will replace my daily snack of potato chips with popcorn or a piece of fruit" or "I will put my fork down between bites."

2 **A SMART goal is measurable.** Unless you have something to measure, it's tough to evaluate your child's success with any degree of accuracy. Here's a measurable goal to increase physical activity: "I'm going to walk three times for 30 minutes this week. Next week, I'll add a 5-minute stretch after each session." There's no doubt about whether or not you meet this goal because it's measurable.

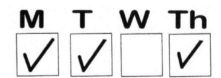

3 **A SMART goal is attainable.** To be sure, you must be able to achieve a goal using the resources available to you right now. For example, a goal aimed at serving your kids a wide variety of fresh fruits for after-school snacks may be difficult or even unattainable during those months when the selection is limited. But, a minor tweak that broadens your goal to include frozen fruits would make it more attainable throughout the year.

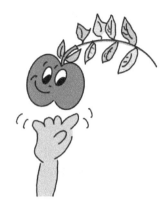

4 **A SMART goal is realistic.** With every goal you set, you should be willing to put in the effort needed to get out of your comfort zone, but don't overdo it. Goals that are too difficult are not only unrealistic, they can be downright frustrating. On the other hand, goals that are too easy typically lead to boredom. Realistic goals have just the right amount of challenge that fuels an "I can do this" attitude.

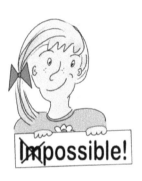

5 **A SMART goal is time sensitive.** Setting the deadline when you expect to achieve a goal is essential for success. Without establishing the time frame in which you expect to accomplish your goal—a meal, a day, a week—your goal is only a dream, and you're likely to travel down the "I'll do it tomorrow" road to failure. Of course, a deadline is also the perfect opportunity to evaluate your progress.

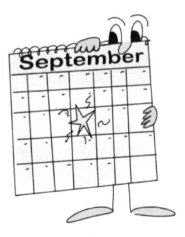

Go for the Goal

To make it easier for you and your family, we have included suggested SMART goals for each month at the end of each chapter. These 12 goals represent a solid foundation for optimal physical and mental health. Meet these goals and your child's active mind and body will be nourished with the high-octane fuel that only sound nutrition can deliver. Inspired to do even more? You'll find "Extra Credit" goals in each chapter to create even more healthy habits.

Before you start, we encourage you to give some serious thought about what you and your child really want to accomplish this year. The more thought you put into setting SMART goals, the better you'll help your child succeed. And, for easier goal tracking, you'll find plenty of **My Smart Tracker** forms in **Chapter 14: Go for the Goal** ready and waiting for you to track your success. Let's get started!

Part 2

Fall Days

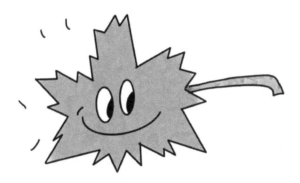

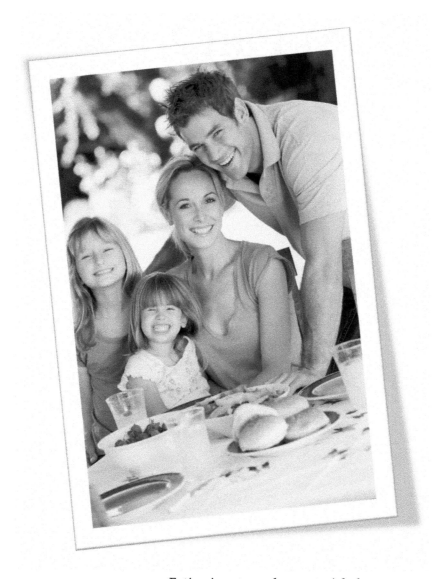

Eating is not merely a material pleasure.
Eating well gives a spectacular joy to life and contributes
immensely to goodwill and happy companionship.
It is of great importance to the morale.
— Elsa Schiaparelli

Chapter 2

September – Family Meals

For most children, September kicks off a new school year, and the new routine is a perfect time to focus on happy and healthy family meals. In fact, of all the healthy behaviors worth making a regular habit, few are more important for boosting your little one's brainpower than sitting down together to enjoy a healthy meal and engaging conversation.

Child development experts agree: Make the family meal a regular habit, and children are more likely to grow up happier, healthier and well-adjusted. They're also more likely to eat fruits, vegetables and other nutrient-rich foods and less likely to drink sugary soft drinks and other empty-calorie foods.

Trouble is, for many parents of young children, September also brings daily schedules that border on superhuman. Alarm clocks are set earlier for the new morning routine. Shuttling the kids to and from school, sports activities, music, dance and art lessons becomes a full-time job. And, motivating their active minds to start—and finish—homework becomes a nightly ritual. That's on top of an already hectic work day. With today's jam-packed schedules, it's easy to see how the family meal can fall by the wayside.

The good news is, you can reclaim your family meals. It's easier than you may think and well worth the effort. After all, shaping the healthy habit of regular family meals is not only linked to better academic performance, but it also helps keep your kids out of trouble.

As younger kids become pre-teens and teenagers, sitting down to frequent family dinners becomes a protective factor that helps curtail a wide variety of high-risk behaviors, according to one study published in *Canadian Family Physician*.[1] In this systematic review, consisting of 14 studies and more than 145,000 children and adolescents, researchers found a consistent link between frequent family meals and a reduced risk of substance abuse, depression or suicidal thoughts, eating disorders and violence. Plus, the researchers reported an increase in self-esteem, grade point averages and commitment to learning.

Family meals are also linked to stronger family bonds and better diet quality. What's more, families that eat regular family meals tend to maintain leaner, healthier body weights. Ready to get started? Read on for the need-to-know essentials to make brain-boosting family meals part of your daily routine.

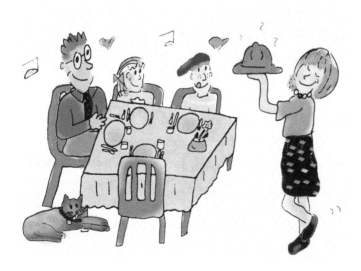

10 Easy Steps for Great Family Meals

1 **Aim for five family meals each week.** With today's hectic, overscheduled lifestyles, the challenge for most families is to make the family meal the rule rather than the exception. Researchers recommend sitting down to an enjoyable family meal at least five times a week. That's the number of occurrences found to have the most positive impact on a child's health and well-being. Start tracking how many times your family eats together. If it's less than five times each week, focus on adding one meal per week until you achieve this goal. If your family sits down to at least five family meals each week, congratulate yourself. You're on track!

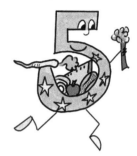

2 **Plan to eat together.** The most common barrier to family meals is busy or conflicting schedules, especially when parents have work schedules that allow little flexibility and kids have activities with strict attendance requirements. The solution is to treat family meals like any other important appointment. Find your calendar now, and schedule your family meals. Remember, aim for at least five per week to be sure you keep this important commitment.

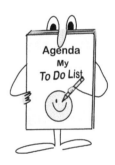

3 **Choose solutions that fit your schedule.** If you can't avoid scheduling sports practice, dance classes or other activities for the kids during your typical dinner hour, plan a simple tailgate or bleacher dinner before practice. Remember, you don't need to cook from scratch, dine at a fancy table or eat off of the good dishes. You just need to eat a healthy meal and enjoy each other's company. If dinner is a challenge due to work schedules, consider scheduling regular family breakfasts to achieve your goal of at least five family meals each week. A Sunday morning family breakfast is an ideal, relaxing option. Get the kids involved. You may be surprised at their creative solutions.

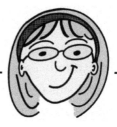

Did You Know?

September is National Family Meals Month. This national initiative was developed to remind parents that the one thing kids really want at the dinner table is you. Here are some tips for success:

- Plan your meals ahead of time.
- Schedule a set time for meals.
- Involve all family members in meal prep and/or clean up.
- Turn off your television and other electronics.
- Focus on the positive; leave the discipline for another time.

4 **Avoid using food as bribes or rewards.** This rule is especially true for younger children. "Eat your peas, and you can have ice cream," may earn you a few bites from your 5-year-old, but it's unlikely to encourage your child to ask for peas again. This type of bribe may seem harmless, but it actually teaches kids to associate certain foods with rewards. Trouble is, these "reward" foods are typically high in fat and sugar and low in brain-building nutrients.

5 **Avoid rushing.** Allow plenty of time to enjoy a family meal that's relaxing. Aim for at least 30 minutes. Rushing reinforces two not-so-good habits: eating too fast and eating too much. This can lead to upset tummies after a meal and excess weight gain over the long run.

6 **Have patience with manners.** Remind your kids to mind their manners, but avoid being too rigid. Use our 1:2 Rule: For every manner in need of reminding—"Elbows off the table," "Sit up straight," "Don't slurp," "Use your fork," "Don't talk with your mouth full"—praise your kids for two they did without reminding.

7 **Create a welcoming experience.** The family meal is more than just about serving healthy foods; it's also about creating an enjoyable, relaxed, welcoming experience. No need to break the bank. Convenient, inexpensive solutions are everywhere from candles or flowers for the table to colorful plates or placemats to cheerful napkins. Your special touch is sure to make family meals more welcoming. And, if kids look forward to a family meal, they're more likely to be open to eating their favorite healthy foods and more likely to try new ones.

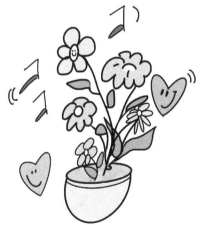

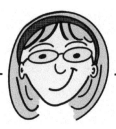

Did You Know?

Sitting down to frequent family meals gives your kids an edge in ways that may surprise you. Here are just a few of the advantages of regular family meals:

- Stronger family ties
- More nutritious diet
- Healthier body weight
- Less substance abuse and other high-risk behaviors

Researchers recommend you aim for at least five family meals each week. Don't forget, all meals count.

8 **Unplug for 30 minutes.** Turn the TV off, banish electronic games during the meal, let voicemail pick up phone calls and focus on conversation. With the typical meal lasting about 30 minutes, unplugging during mealtime is doable even for the most sophisticated techies among us—kids and adults alike.

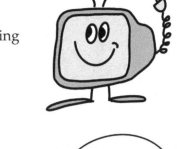

9 **Talk it up.** Engage everyone in conversation. Talking, not the food, should be the focus. Keep the conversation positive, encouraging and upbeat. Focus on positive topics such as "What did you do today to make it a good day?" Avoid arguments and save potentially stressful subjects for a non-meal time.

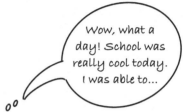

Wow, what a day! School was really cool today. I was able to...

10 **Banish the clean plate club.** If your child refuses to eat broccoli, don't pressure and don't make a big deal about it. Be sure to offer it again at another meal, perhaps at several meals, but avoid pressure. Remember, your goal is to offer nutritious foods frequently enough so your kids have many opportunities to choose them.

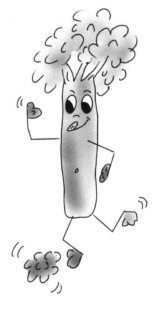

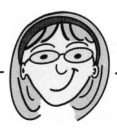

Did You Know?

You can teach your kids a smarter way to use their homework time. Here's how: Simply decide on the amount of time to spend on each subject before your child starts. For example, if your daughter has 45 minutes to tackle her homework, she could decide to spend 20 minutes on algebra, 15 minutes on language and 10 minutes to review for a spelling test. Not only do kids learn a valuable lesson in budgeting their time, but they'll use that time more efficiently.

What's for Dinner?

For most families, dinner is the best time for family meals. Don't worry, it doesn't have to be complicated or time consuming. It doesn't even have to be home cooked. Simple, delicious meals planned together are the best.

Get the family involved by allowing each person to choose a favorite menu for at least one meal each week. Even young children have a favorite main dish, vegetable and fruit to plan a meal around. Keep things interesting by occasionally adding a new food for the family to try. You never know when you'll stumble on a new favorite.

When you plan and schedule family meals, you'll also reap the benefits that anticipation provides. When kids know when and what to expect for the meal, they feel more secure, avoid grazing on junk food before the meal and come to the table hungry, but not starving. In this way, your kids will be able to better enjoy the nutritious foods you serve.

> ### Parent Pearl
>
> **Set an appreciation plate.** As a family, we sometimes set a special place setting at the dinner table to spotlight one family member. During the meal, each person shares what they appreciate about the mealtime star. Everyone benefits from the feel-good nature of positive sharing.

Don't Forget Breakfast

As mentioned above, breakfast can be another opportunity for a family meal. What's more, eating a healthy breakfast gets your child's day started off on the right foot and nourishes active learning. Shape this healthy behavior when your kids are young, and they'll be more likely to make it a daily habit as they age.

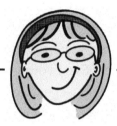

Did You Know?

Looking for a quick and brainy tailgate meal? Here are five no-fuss ideas to try:

1. A thermos of soup with a hearty whole grain roll.
2. Sandwich fixings packed in a pita pocket.
3. Ready-made rotisserie chicken with a pre-packed salad.
4. An upgraded peanut butter and jelly sandwich. Add sliced banana, cut into finger-sized portions and serve with sliced oranges, grapes, strawberries or other small fruits.
5. Whole grain crackers with hummus or sliced cheese and luncheon meats with a fruit salad.

For those mornings when your routine is already jam-packed, a ready-in-minutes breakfast is ideal to fuel hungry minds with essential nutrients for learning. A hot bowl of oatmeal with fruit and nuts, whole wheat toast topped with peanut butter and applesauce or whole grain toaster waffles with fresh fruit and a glass of milk are just a few no-fuss solutions to start the day right.

Meal Time is Multi Time

Be sure to fill any potential nutrient gap between what your child is eating and what their growing body and active brain actually need with a daily multivitamin.

High-quality multivitamins designed to please even the most finicky kids are readily available from squishy gummies and chewable cartoon characters to flavored liquids and sour tarts. Choose your favorite, but make sure it's a complete multivitamin developed just for kids to ensure the proper amount of essential nutrients.

A word about iron. Iron is the most common nutrient deficiency among children, yet it's critical for learning. Nutrition experts recommend that young children, age 4 to 8 years, consume at least 10 milligrams of iron per day. Older kids, age 9 to 13 years, should consume at least 8 milligrams of iron per day. A kid's multi that includes a little iron is a great way to help ensure your child gets enough of this important nutrient for everyday learning.

> **Parent Pearl**
>
> **Whip up a healthy breakfast.** My kids gobble up my fast-scrambled eggs. I beat two eggs together with ¼ cup milk in a microwave-safe dish and microwave for about 2 minutes. It rises like a soufflé. Fluff with a fork and sprinkle with cheese. I serve with whole wheat toast topped with avocado, fresh fruit and milk, and the kids are ready to start their day.

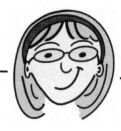

Did You Know?

Multivitamins are easier on the stomach and better absorbed when taken with food. So, encourage your child to take a multi with a meal—every day.

By giving your child a complete multivitamin every day, you help guard against food jags, finicky eating and half-eaten lunches. It's a type of dietary insurance that helps ensure your child is getting the nutrients needed to stay focused and sharp all day long.

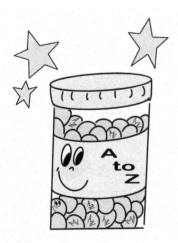

Once you've found a favorite, shape a regular habit so your child remembers to take their multi every day. We recommend taking a daily multi at breakfast. It's an easy routine to get into, it fuels the day with added nutrition, and it's one less thing you need to think about for the rest of the day.

Choosing a quality multivitamin

With so many choices, shopping for a kid's multivitamin can be confusing. Here are a few tips to make it easier to spot a quality product:

- **Choose a multi formulated for kids.** This helps ensure the amount of each nutrient aligns with your child's needs. Plus, a kid-friendly flavor makes it easier to shape a daily habit.
- **Look for a quality mark.** Check labels for trusted names in third-party quality testing like NSF International, United States Pharmacopeia (USP) or ConsumerLab.com.
- **Choose a complete multi.** A "complete" multi ensures a full complement of essential vitamins and minerals, including some iron and calcium, two nutrients that tend to fall short in a kid's diet.
- **Avoid undesirable ingredients.** Read labels to avoid high fructose corn syrup, artificial sweeteners, flavors and colors and other undesirable ingredients.
- **Look beyond vitamins and minerals.** Omega-3 fatty acids and phytonutrients like anthocyanins, lycopene or lutein provide a beneficial nutrient bonus.
- **Buy enough, but not too much.** Buy a bottle size that you can use before the expiration date on the label when vitamins begin to degrade.

A word of caution

Store products out of reach of young children. Accidental overdose of iron-containing products is a leading cause of fatal poisoning in children under 6 years. Talk to older kids and remind them that a multi is not a candy. Don't exceed the suggested use unless directed by your child's pediatrician.

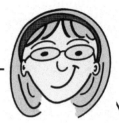

Did You Know?

When it comes to the number of family members at your dinner table, as few as two members count. Why? The main goal is adequate time to connect and converse. Need inspiration? Here are a few conversation starters from the non-profit Family Dinner Project:

- What is the best thing that happened to you today?
- If you could have any superpower, what would it be? How would you use it to help people or make this a better world?
- Choose a job you love, and you will never have to work a day in your life. What do you think this means? (ages 8-13 y)

For additional conversation starters, recipes and more, consider joining The Family Dinner Project, a nonprofit initiative started by Harvard fellow Shelly London in 2010. This online community is now a movement that advances and champions the benefits of eating together as a family. Who doesn't love that? Learn more at https://thefamilydinnerproject.org.

TV Advertising & Brain Drain

It's no surprise that brain-building foods typically fail to top the list of foods and beverages advertised to children on television. In fact, it's just the opposite. Food advertising to young children continues to entice them to eat high-fat, sugary, salty foods and beverages with little or no nutritional value.

Some major food and beverage companies have pledged to market only healthier foods to children as part of the Better Business Bureau's Children's Food and Beverage Advertising Initiative. However, the pledge is often not upheld. In fact, a whopping 88% of advertisements by companies taking the pledge continue to promote unhealthy foods to kids, according to one study.[2] So much for good intentions.

Adding insult to injury is the fact that advertising to children now extends beyond television to internet sites and social media platforms, not to mention a seemingly endless number of mobile apps.[3] Not only are kids willing to break their own piggy banks to buy the latest advertised brand, but they'll also want you to empty your wallet to buy it for them. Researchers call this "influencing purchases and requests to buy." Parents know it as that all too familiar—and entirely too persistent—must-have-it nagging. This advertising power is especially troublesome for younger children, who typically have difficulty understanding the persuasive intent of unhealthy food advertising.[4]

> **Parent Pearl**
>
> **At breakfast, we use the cereal box to inspire a few brainteasers.** How many adjectives start with the letter "S"? How much calcium is in one serving? What do you think inspired the name of the cereal? It's a great way to foster my child's reading and critical thinking skills.

To be sure, an occasional treat won't harm your child's growing brain, but the daily nagging can certainly chip away at your resolve to keep the amount of junk food in your child's diet to a minimum. The good news is research suggests that all this advertising only moderately affects a young child's beliefs about foods and beverages and their typical dietary intake. For the most part, the influence of television advertising on young children is limited to short-term consumption. So, your challenge is to keep the whining at bay, while instilling healthy habits and food choices.

Parent Pearl

Schedule routine eye exams. Our pediatrician always mentions how important good eyesight is for optimal learning. So, I make sure I schedule a complete eye exam for each of my kids as part of our annual back-to-school preparations.

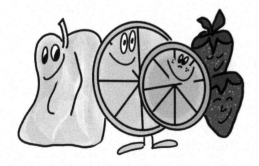

Simple Ways to Fight TV Advertising

1 **Be a good role model.** When it comes to shaping healthy habits in your kids, your actions speak volumes.

2 **Limit screen time.** This is especially true for commercial programming. However, guidelines for television watching have become murky. At one time, the American Academy of Pediatrics (AAP) recommended kids limit TV watching to no more than 2 hours per day. However, today kids are exposed to so many more screens—computer, tablet, smart phones—and many of them offer educational benefits. For this reason, AAP recognized it's tough to set a one-number-fits-all approach. Instead, the key is to ensure your child is leading a balanced life, sleeping well, socializing with friends, reading, creating, and overall feeling positive. To help you create a plan that's right for your child and family, the AAP has developed the Media Use Plan. For all the details, visit http://healthychildren.org/MediaUsePlan.[5]

3 **Choose programming on non-commercial stations whenever possible.** This will help reduce exposure to ads for high-fat, sugary foods.

4 **Discuss marketing techniques with your kids.** This will help your children understand the persuasive intent of ads.

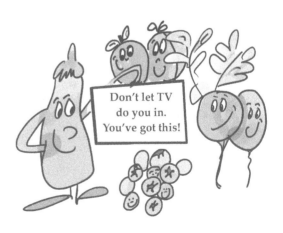

12 Quick & Brainy After-School Snacks

1. Apple slices dipped in almond butter (or other favorite type of nut butter)
2. Edamame
3. Fresh fruit (in season)
4. Hummus with pita bread and/or veggies
5. Macaroni & cheese
6. Popcorn
7. Pretzels
8. Pumpkin bread
9. Quesadilla or grilled cheese sandwich (with whole wheat tortilla or bread, respectively)
10. Smoothie
11. String cheese
12. Walnuts and raisins, smoked almonds or your child's favorite trail mix-style combination

Parent Pearl

Routine can rock. Have your child put any special school projects and all homework in their backpack the night before and place it by the door. This simple routine helps prevent the forgetfulness that can occur during the morning dash out the door.

This Month's Smart Goal

I will add one family meal each week to reach at least five per week.*

*At least five is the goal, but for this goal and all others, start where you and your family are. A goal shouldn't be too hard (or too easy).

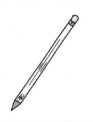

This Month's Extra Credit

I will give my child a children's multivitamin with iron every day, preferably at breakfast.

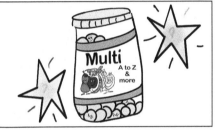

To monitor your daily progress toward your goals, use the **My Smart Tracker** forms in **Chapter 14: Go for the Goal.**

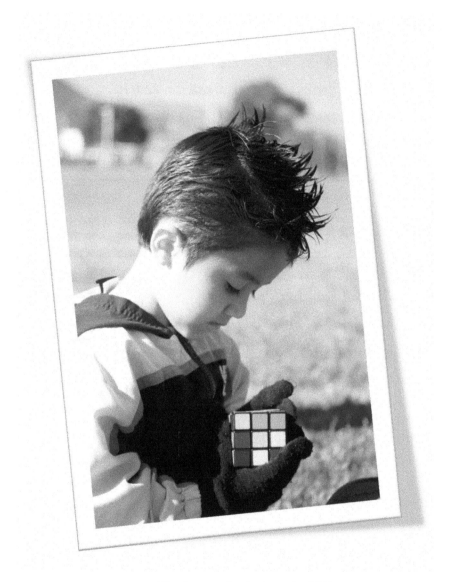

The human brain has 100 billion neurons,
each neuron connected to 10 thousand other
neurons. Sitting on your shoulders is the most
complicated object in the known universe.
— Dr. Michio Kaku, PhD

Chapter 3

October – Feed a Growing Brain

Of all the advantages you can give your child to help them excel, nourishing their brain ranks among the most important. After all, when the brain is well-nourished, focused attention, eager learning and excellent grades are sure to follow. In this chapter, you'll learn what to look for when choosing the best brain foods for your rising star.

Foods that Activate Nerve Cells

Nerve cells (or neurons) communicate using a variety of biochemical messengers called neurotransmitters. The signal starts when one neuron sends out a neurotransmitter to a neighboring neuron to spark it into action. The neighboring neuron does the same to its neighbor and so on. The signaling continues over a vast neural network that would rival the most complex metropolitan freeway system.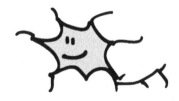

To make these important neurotransmitters, the body needs a steady supply of foods that contain protein. Why? Protein contains nitrogen-based compounds called amino acids, including the so-called essential amino acids that must be provided in the diet because the body can't make them. Many amino acids, including some of the essential ones, serve as building blocks for the body's production of neurotransmitters critical for learning and other mental functions.

How much protein does your child need for optimal learning? Aim for at least 19 grams of protein per day for young kids, age 4 to 8 years, and at least 34 grams per day for older children, age 9 to 13 years.

The good news is many protein-rich foods are also kid-friendly foods, making it even easier to prepare nourishing meals and snacks. Read on for our top brain-boosting, protein-rich food choices.

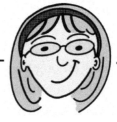

Did You Know?

You've probably heard the adage, "Breakfast is the most important meal of the day." We couldn't agree more.

The serious benefits of breakfast are revealed in one systematic review of 26 studies. Here, researchers found eating breakfast was directly linked to better mental performance, academic success, quality of life and overall wellbeing. Results are published in the September 2019 issue of *Food & Nutrition Research*.[1] When it comes to what to serve for breakfast, think variety, starting with nutrient-rich whole grains, fruits and vegetables, and protein-rich foods. Bon appetite!

Protein-Rich Brain Foods

1 **Milk.** Each 1-cup serving provides **about 8 grams** of brain-boosting protein. Dairy milk is the kid-friendly option, but don't overlook plant-based milk beverages like fortified soy milk that provide **about 6 to 8 grams** of protein per serving. If you have a picky eater, whole milk and its rich flavor may help entice your child to drink up. On the other hand, if your child tends to be on the heavier side, it's best to fill the fridge with low-fat or fat-free milk products.[2] These options are still packed with protein and other nutrients for active brains, just without the extra calories.

2 **Yogurt**. Each 6-ounce serving provides **about 8 grams** of protein. Like milk, low-fat varieties are available, and many brands offer delicious natural flavors without added sugars. You're sure to find a few that will make your little genius smile. Better yet, serve up creamy plain Greek yogurt with a scoop of naturally sweet berries or other fruit.

3 **Cheese**. Each 1-ounce serving provides **about 7 grams**, so it's hard to beat cheese for a protein boost. The next time you serve up a warm bowl of macaroni and cheese, a grilled cheese sandwich or other cheesy favorite, remember the brain-boosting benefits of cheese.

4 **Lean Meat, Fish and Poultry.** From lean hamburgers to fish fillets to grilled chicken, these protein-rich foods boast **about 7 grams** of protein per ounce. Aim for healthy portions (about 2 ounces per meal or the size of two ping pong balls).

Parent Pearl

My on-the-go kids love trail mix with almonds, cashews and other nuts. Each week, I make a big batch and portion it out into single-serving, reusable bags. It's an easy-to-grab, protein-rich snack that also keeps hundreds of disposable baggies out of the landfill.

5 **Dried Beans, Peas and Lentils.** Kidney, navy, garbanzo and other dried beans as well as split green peas and hearty lentils are inexpensive nutrient wonders that pack **about 7 to 9 grams** of protein in each one-half cup serving. A warm bowl of chili, baked beans or other hearty bean dish is perfect for brisk October days.

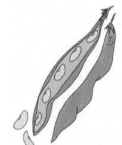

6 **Eggs.** Each egg provides **about 7 grams** of protein making it an ideal protein choice. Serve them scrambled, poached over fiber-rich, whole-wheat toast, in a cheese omelet, or hard-boiled for the lunch box.

7 **Peanut Butter.** Peanut butter provides **about 4 grams** of protein per 1-tablespoon serving. Offer a hearty PB&J on 100% whole grain bread, a celery boat stuffed with peanut butter or the occasional peanut butter cookie. For kids who don't like peanut butter, consider a nut butter made with almonds, cashews or other tree nuts. These provide **about 3 to 4 grams** of protein per 1-tablespoon serving. Although, if your child has a peanut allergy, talk to your pediatrician before using any other nut butter.

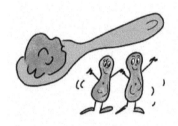

8 **Nuts and Seeds.** Almonds, cashews, peanuts, walnuts and other nuts provide between **4 to 7 grams** of protein per 1-ounce serving (about 10 to 20 nuts, depending on the variety). Nuts are high in calories, so be sure to keep the serving size in check. Consider buying nuts and seeds in bulk, then portioning them out in single-serving, reusable containers for on-the-go activities, lunch boxes and snacks.

9 **Whole Grains.** While not the protein powerhouse of other food groups, whole grain foods—brown rice, whole grain pasta, whole wheat bread and others—are still good sources with **about 3 grams** of protein per one-half cup or 1-ounce serving.

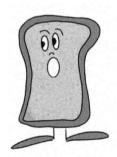

Foods that Shape Up Brain Cells

One of the hallmarks of a healthy cell is a pliable, flexible membrane ready and able to drink in nutrients needed for peak performance and eliminate toxins and metabolic byproducts that may cause harm. Your child's brain cells are no exception and will thrive when nourished by a nutrient-rich diet.

You can help prime your child's brain cells for optimal learning by focusing on two key nutrients essential for healthy cell membranes not only in the brain, but throughout the body. These nutrients are choline and omega-3 essential fatty acids.

Choline

Choline is a chemical cousin to the vitamin B family. It serves as a building block for phosphatidylcholine, sometimes referred to as lecithin. This fat-like compound wiggles its way into the membranes that surround cells, including brain cells. Here, it not only fortifies the structural integrity of the cell membrane, which helps control the flow of materials into and out of a cell, but also plays quarterback in the chemical signaling that triggers cells into action.

The body also uses choline to synthesize acetylcholine, a chemical messenger in the brain that's critical for cell-to-cell communication involved in learning, memory and other functions. Nutrition experts recommend that young children, age 4 to 8 years, consume at least 250 milligrams of choline per day, but avoid exceeding 1,000 milligrams per day. Older kids, age 9 to 13 years, should consume at least 375 milligrams of choline per day, but avoid exceeding 2,000 milligrams per day.[3]

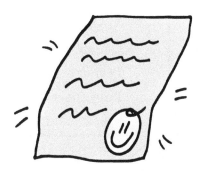

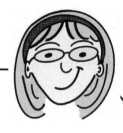

Did You Know?

Your child needs to consume choline every day to nourish their growing brain for optimal mental performance. Young kids (age 4 to 8 years) need at least 250 milligrams every day. Older kids (age 9 to 13 years) need at least 375 milligrams every day. The good news is choline is found in many kid-friendly foods.

Food (Serving Size)	Choline (milligrams)
Egg (1 large)	100 mg
Fish filet, cod (3 ounces)	71 mg
Hamburger (3 ounces)	64 mg
Chicken breast (3 ounces)	62 mg
Soymilk (1 cup)	58 mg
Soybeans, cooked (½ cup)	41 mg
Milk, 2% low-fat (1 cup)	40 mg
Milk, whole (1 cup)	35 mg
Broccoli, cooked (½ cup)	31 mg
Kidney beans, cooked (½ cup)	27 mg
Yogurt, regular (6 ounces)	26 mg
Cauliflower, cooked (½ cup)	24 mg
Peanut butter, chunky (2 tablespoons)	20 mg
Peas, cooked (½ cup)	14 mg
Wheat germ (1 tablespoon)	13 mg

Source: USDA FoodData Central (https://fdc.nal.usda.gov).

Food sources of choline

Choline is widely distributed in foods, but the most common kid-friendly foods are egg yolks and milk. One large egg provides about 100 milligrams of choline, and one cup of milk provides about 35 to 40 milligrams of choline. But don't overlook other sources of choline your child may enjoy such as foods made with soybeans, beef, fish, chicken, peanuts or vegetables such as broccoli and cauliflower.

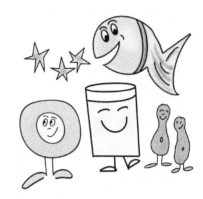

Omega-3 Fatty Acids

Omega-3 fatty acids (also known as omega-3 fats) are among the largest fatty acids in the body. They sit on chemical backbones ranging from 18 to 22 carbon molecules, which is Goliath in biochemical terms.

When it comes to brain health, two omega-3 fatty acids—ALA (alpha-linolenic acid) and EPA (eicosapentaenoic acid)—can lend a helping hand, but the star is DHA (docosahexaenoic acid).[4] We must consume ALA in the foods we eat because our bodies can't make it. In the body, ALA can be converted into EPA and finally into DHA with the help of a few enzymes. These are important conversion steps because both EPA and DHA influence the structure of cell membranes and function of cells, while DHA plays an important structural role in the eye and brain. Trouble is, the rate of conversion is less than impressive. In fact, some researchers report the body converts less than 10% of the typical ALA intake into EPA and DHA.[5]

If we eat enough DHA-rich foods, we don't need to rely on the body's meager ability to convert ALA to DHA. Sadly though, the typical American diet doesn't come close to providing an adequate intake. For example, health experts around the world recommend a daily intake of EPA and DHA combined in the range of 200 to 500 milligrams.[6] Yet, most American children fail to meet even the lowest recommended intake for these fatty acids.[7]

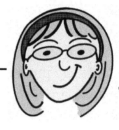

Did You Know?

Walnuts, flaxseed and certain vegetable oils are some of the richest food sources of ALA (alpha-linolenic acid). Cold-water fish such as salmon, sardines and tuna are one of the best food sources of the longer chain omega-3 fatty acids EPA (eicosapentaenoic acid) and DHA (docosahexaenoic acid).

Food	Omega-3 Fatty Acid (milligrams)	
	ALA	EPA + DHA
Walnuts, English (14 halves)	2,570 mg	--
Flaxseed oil (1 teaspoon)	2,420 mg	--
Flaxseed, ground (1 teaspoon)	570 mg	--
Canola oil (1 teaspoon)	350 mg	--
Soybean oil (1 teaspoon)	308 mg	--
Sardines, canned in oil (2 each)	120 mg	230 mg
Spinach, cooked (½ cup)	82 mg	--
Salmon, cooked (3 ounces)	50 mg	340 mg
Olive oil (1 teaspoon)	34 mg	--
Tuna, canned in water (3 ounces)	3 mg	192 mg

Source: USDA FoodData Central (https://fdc.nal.usda.gov).

Food sources of omega-3 fats

What foods are good sources of omega-3 fatty acids? English walnuts, flaxseed, green leafy vegetables such as purslane and spinach and certain vegetable oils—canola, soybean, flaxseed, linseed and olive—are particularly good food sources of ALA. Fish, particularly cold-water fish such as salmon, haddock, mackerel, tuna, anchovies and sardines, contain high amounts of EPA and DHA. In addition, manufacturers add these brain-boosting fats to packaged foods such as orange juice and eggs, so it's worth comparing labels to choose a brand fortified with omega-3's.

> **Parent Pearl**
>
> **I give my kids a fish oil supplement every day.** It's an easy way to help ensure they're getting enough brain-building omega-3 DHA. To entice them, I buy a brand with a natural fruit flavor.

Don't overlook dietary supplements with omega-3 fats. These help fill any potential nutrient gap between what your child gets in the foods they eat and what their body needs. Fish and krill oils are common marine sources of omega-3 supplements. Algal oil sources are available too, which is a welcome option for vegans, vegetarians and those who prefer to avoid fishy burps.

A word of caution

While fish is a great source of DHA, the brain-boosting omega-3 fatty acid, some types—shark, swordfish, king mackerel and tilefish—tend to concentrate higher amounts of the toxic heavy metal mercury. What's a parent to do? Start by choosing fish known to be lower in mercury more often. Think shellfish, canned fish, smaller ocean fish and farm-raised fish. Next, choose a supplement that meets strict quality standards for low mercury content.

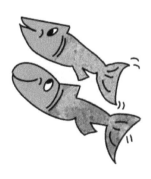

Foods that Protect Brain Cells

A diet rich in lutein may also provide the mental juice your child needs to excel in the classroom. Why? While nutrition experts recognize lutein for its eye health benefits, its potential to protect the brain and support cognitive function may be even more impressive, especially for children.[8]

Lutein is a yellow carotenoid found in many colorful fruits and vegetables. It's one of two carotenoids found in the human eye. The other is lutein's chemical cousin zeaxanthin. Once absorbed in the intestine, lutein and zeaxanthin travel through the bloodstream protected by fat-loving lipoproteins (carotenoids don't like watery solutions like blood) and then deposit in the retina. They have a particular affinity for the macula lutea (the central area of the retina essential for sharp, central vision), which they saturate with their protective yellow pigment.

Lutein and better eye health

To say your eyes prefer these two carotenoids would be an understatement. They are the only carotenoids able to cross the blood-retina barrier,[9] and they do so in a big way. Lutein, in particular, has been reported to reach a concentration in the macula that's as much as 1,000 times higher than that in the blood.[10]

In the eye, lutein not only works as a powerful antioxidant, it also helps filter out high-energy blue light that can damage photoreceptors in the retina and cause eyestrain that can make it difficult for a child to concentrate. Sunlight is a common source of harmful blue light. Another culprit is electronic devices with screens that emit blue light, devices like cell phones, tablets and computers. It's a modern-day challenge for children who may spend several hours a day staring into these screens both at school and at home. It's also a big reason a lutein-rich diet can go a long way to help protect a child's vision and eye health.

Lutein and better mental function

Emerging research shows lutein is the major carotenoid throughout the entire human brain, including areas that control mental function. Researchers have yet to fully understand why the brain is equipped to drink in so much lutein. What they do know is lutein is the only carotenoid consistently linked with a wide range of cognitive functions, including language, learning and memory.

In fact, some researchers believe that lutein may have a special neuroprotective role in young kids. In one clinical study,[11] young school-aged children who had higher macular pigment density (a biomarker for brain lutein) were able to complete a standardized cognitive task with less brain activation and significantly fewer mistakes than children who had lower macular pigment density. In other words, they needed less brain power to perform better on a demanding mental task that required them to process information and pay attention.

Lutein and better antioxidant protection

The same powerful antioxidant action that lutein exerts to protect the retina may also play a role in the brain. Why? Not only do brain cells have an especially high fatty acid content, they also have a high metabolic activity. That's a double whammy that makes neurons vulnerable to attack by unstable free radicals. For this reason, a regular intake of lutein-rich foods is just what your child's active brain needs.

A recommended dietary intake for lutein and zeaxanthin has yet to be determined. Some of the best food sources are spinach, kale and other dark green, leafy vegetables, but don't overlook other colorful fruits and vegetables and egg yolks. You'll also find carotenoids in high-quality dietary supplements specifically formulated for children to support brain and vision health.

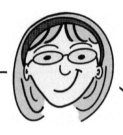

Did You Know?

Dark green, leafy vegetables are a rich source of lutein and zeaxanthin, but other colorful fruits and vegetables and egg yolks are good sources too. Choose a variety to add to your child's daily plate to protect both brain and eye health.

Food (Serving Size)	Lutein & Zeaxanthin (milligrams)
Kale, cooked (½ cup)	11.8
Spinach, cooked (½ cup)	10.1
Spinach, raw (1 cup)	3.0
Peas, cooked (½ cup)	1.9
Kale, raw (1 cup)	1.3
Yellow squash, sliced (½ cup)	1.2
Brussel sprouts, cooked (½ cup)	1.0
Corn, cooked (½ cup)	0.7
Broccoli, chopped, cooked (½ cup)	0.5
Egg (1 large)	0.5
Avocado, raw, cubes (½ cup)	0.2
Sweet green pepper, sliced (½ cup)	0.2
Grapes (1 cup)	0.1
Orange juice (½ cup)	0.1

Source: USDA FoodData Central (https://fdc.nal.usda.gov).

Foods that Nourish the Gut-Brain Axis

The health of your child's brain depends on the constant biochemical cross-talk that occurs between their gut bacteria and their brain. It's called the gut-brain axis, and it relies on a wide variety of biochemical pathways (neural, endocrine, immune and metabolic) to help regulate the central nervous system and maintain peak performance.[13] As you may have guessed, it all starts with a healthy gut microbiome.

In the simplest terms, the gut microbiome is the collection of all the bacteria that reside in the digestive tract, mostly in the large intestine. But there's nothing simple about it. In fact, some experts call the gut microbiome the most densely populated microbial ecosystem on the planet. It includes both health-promoting "good" bacteria and disease-causing "bad" bacteria. Some bacteria stick to the cells that line the intestinal wall where they mostly fortify immune defenses. Others travel freely through the intestine and eventually end up in the stool. But before they do, these microscopic critters perform some amazing nutritional feats.

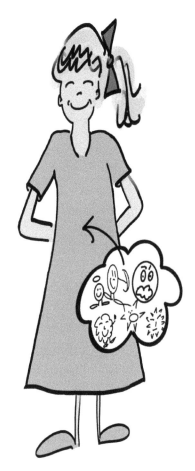

Gut bacteria in action

Gut bacteria have unique enzymes that break down chemical bonds that human digestive enzymes can't. In this way, they play a key role in breaking down carbohydrates, proteins and other food components that reach the large intestine undigested. Gut bacteria also produce short-chain fatty acids that not only provide energy, but help activate numerous biochemical pathways throughout the body. And, they even synthesize essential vitamins like vitamin B12 and vitamin K.[14]

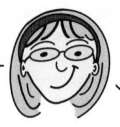

Did You Know?

In the gut, prebiotic fibers deliver a wide range of health benefits beyond brain health. Here are eight more reasons to fill your child's plate with prebiotic-rich fruits, vegetables, nuts, seeds, grains and legumes. Prebiotic fibers help:[15]

1. Promote better intestinal absorption of bone-building calcium.
2. Support the growth of health-promoting bacteria like Bifidobacteria and Lactobacilli.
3. Produce short-chain fatty acids and other health-promoting metabolites.
4. Decrease the production of cancer-causing metabolites from undigested protein.
5. Inhibit the growth of disease-causing bacteria.
6. Reduce the risk of allergies.
7. Fortify the integrity of intestinal cells, which helps block the absorption of toxins.
8. Improve immune defense by influencing the activity of key immune cells.

Each person has a unique makeup of gut bacteria, and it's constantly in flux. Many factors like age, weight, health status, activity level or stress can alter its makeup. The use of medications can play a role, too. Yet, what you eat is the one factor that reigns supreme when it comes to bringing balance and diversity to this important microscopic community.

Nourishing your child's gut bacteria

By far, the best way your child can maintain a healthy gut microbiome is to eat more plant-based foods, every day. Why? These foods are rich in prebiotic fibers that stimulate the growth and activity of health-promoting gut bacteria.

For example, foods like oats, barley, mushrooms and algae contain one type of prebiotic fiber called beta glucans. Onions, chicory, garlic, asparagus, bananas and artichokes contain another type called fructo-oligosaccharides or FOS.[16] And, leeks, asparagus, onions, wheat, garlic, chicory, oats, soybeans and Jerusalem artichokes[15] contain a prebiotic fiber called inulin. These are just a few examples of the many types of prebiotic fibers that naturally occur in plant foods.

Parent Pearl

My kids can be finicky when it comes to eating broccoli and other steamed veggies. So, I garnish with just enough grated cheese for flavor—about 1 teaspoon per serving. It's a delicious, nutrient-rich way to boost their veggie intake.

Keep things simple

Don't worry, there's no need to get bogged down looking for foods with specific types of prebiotic fibers. Instead, simply include a wide variety of plant-based foods in your child's diet such as fruits, vegetables, grains and legumes. Even seeds and nuts contain prebiotic fibers.[17] In this way, you help ensure your child gets enough prebiotic fiber on a regular basis to nourish and maintain a healthy gut microbiome.

Another way to help maintain a healthy gut microbiome is by eating more fermented foods. One strategy is to include a few of these tangy options on the weekly menu. Foods like yogurt, kefir, kimchi or sauerkraut are good choices. Fermented foods are rich sources of probiotics, good bacteria that can help bring balance to the gut microflora. What's more, you see the benefits of these dietary changes in a matter of days.

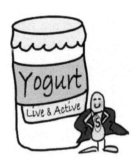

High-Octane Foods

When it comes to fueling your child's brain for focused attention and learning, nothing beats starchy foods. Nutrition experts call these complex carbohydrates. You can call them high-octane fuel for growing brains. Your best bets are starchy foods that are also high in fiber. Think whole grain cereals, breads and pastas as well as brown rice, peas, beans and starchy veggies.

From the first bite, these foods set off a cascade of digestive enzymes that go to work breaking down large starch molecules into simple sugars the body is able to absorb and release into the bloodstream to fuel organs and tissues. One such simple sugar, glucose, is the brain's main energy source.

As the body's most complex organ, the brain demands an enormous amount of energy and requires constant refueling. How do you ensure your child's brain has a steady supply of glucose for learning? It all has to do with keeping their blood sugar level fairly steady throughout the day—not too high and not too low. Some starchy foods work better than others at this. These are known as low-glycemic index foods.

Ranking foods by their GI value

The Glycemic Index (GI for short) is a system that ranks foods based on how they affect blood sugar levels immediately after being consumed. Carbohydrates that are digested slowly have lower GI values. They release glucose into the bloodstream gradually, drip by drip, which helps maintain a steady blood sugar level after you eat them. Examples include milk, whole wheat bread and oatmeal. By contrast,

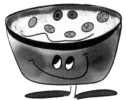

carbohydrates that are digested quickly like white bread, white rice and mashed potatoes have higher GI values. These foods are absorbed quickly and lead to a blood sugar response that can be too fast and too high.

It's a little tricky though, since a food's GI value is affected by the way its prepared, the amount of protein, fat and fiber it contains, and other factors. Refined and sugary foods release their sugar quickly, which can spike blood sugar, so they have higher GI values. By contrast, foods that also contain fiber, fat and protein release sugar more slowly so they have lower GI values. And, since longer cooking times (and chopping) break down food more during prep, these foods release sugars faster which lead to higher GI values. Did we say tricky?

GI foods and brain health

What's the best way to use the GI system to support brain health? No need to banish high-GI foods from your child's diet, just choose them less often or balance them with low-GI foods at the same meal. Whenever possible, serve up low-GI options of carb-rich favorites. Think a stick-to-your-ribs porridge from rolled oats instead of a plain bagel for breakfast. Whole wheat bread instead of white bread for a lunchbox sandwich. Or, nutty brown rice instead of plain white rice for dinner.

Where to learn more

You'll find the GI values of your favorite foods in a searchable database at www.glycemicindex.com. Aim to include more low-GI foods (55 or less) at meals and snacks to help your child maintain healthy blood sugar levels after eating. It's an ideal way to fuel busy brains with energizing glucose from the first morning class to long after homework is done.

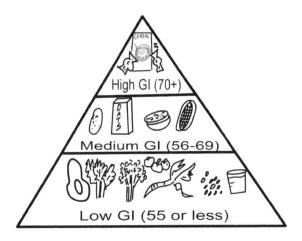

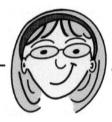

Did You Know?

When consumed alone, foods with a high Glycemic Index (GI) value (70 or above) can lead to a blood sugar response that's too fast and too high. You don't need to completely avoid high GI foods for better blood sugar control. Instead, consume them with foods that have a lower or no GI value at the same meal or snack. Only foods that contain carbohydrates have a GI value. Meat, fish, eggs, avocado and other foods that contain little or no carbs won't have a GI value. In short, no carbs, no GI value.

This Month's Smart Goal

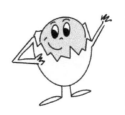

I will serve breakfast every day and include a protein-rich food.

This Month's Extra Credit

I will give my child a DHA supplement every day, preferably at breakfast.

To monitor your daily progress toward your goals, use the **My Smart Tracker** forms in **Chapter 14: Go for the Goal.**

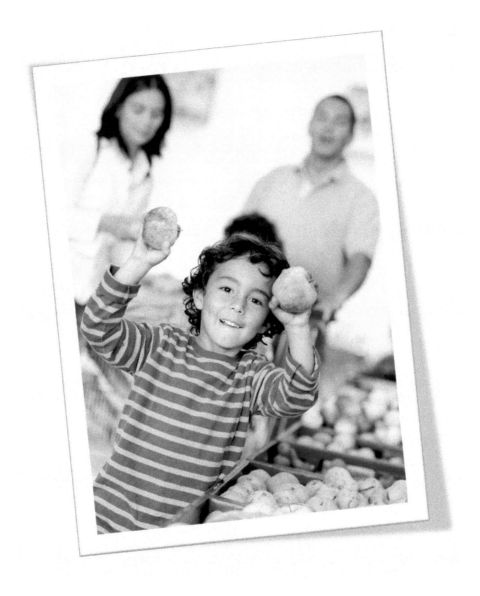

What pleases the eye pleases the body as a whole.
— Deepak Chopra

Chapter 4

November – Eat Your Colors

Mother Nature surrounds us with beautiful colors all year. Think of green leaves transforming into brilliant reds, oranges and yellows as summer fades into autumn, or imagine a rainbow bursting forth after a spring shower. Fruits and vegetables are no exception with a rich color palette with just about every hue imaginable. Think deep purple plums, vibrant red peppers, sunny oranges, crisp green lettuce or bright white cauliflower.

Like many parents, you may not think twice about the color of the produce you feed your child. Yet, helping your child eat a diet rich in colorful fruits and veggies can have a profound impact on overall health, including brain health. In fact, this simple behavior—eating a wide variety of colors—is one of the most significant dietary habits that you can establish to steer your child toward a healthier future while promoting brain health and protecting brain cells from damage.

Why should you focus on serving up meals in living color? In a word: Phytonutrients. Plants produce a wide variety of these bioactive compounds to protect against environmental insults from insect infestations to extreme temperatures to pesticide exposure and beyond.[1,2] When your child eats them, these very same phytonutrients go to work to protect overall health, including brain health.

What's the best way to ensure your child is eating the amount and type of phytonutrients that will protect their brain? Make sure they eat a colorful diet. How? Simply focus on eating fruits and veggies with skin or flesh in the five key color groups every day. These color groups include purple, red, orange-yellow, green and white-brown. The good news is it's easier than you may think, especially after a quick primer on each of these colorful food groups. Read on to get started.

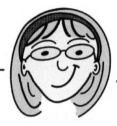

Did You Know?

MyPlate is a national education campaign from the USDA's Center for Nutrition Policy and Promotion. It's a great resource for fun facts and activities to inspire your kids to eat a healthy diet, including fruits and vegetables.

Here, you'll find a wide selection of kid-friendly activities like interactive games and apps, printable activity sheets and other fun ways to teach kids about healthy eating. Best of all, it's free. Make it a family affair and get everyone involved. Learn more at www.myplate.gov.

The Purple Group

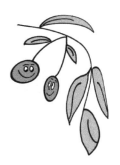

Purple fruits and vegetables come in a variety of shades from the deep violet purple of an eggplant to the purple-red of a beet to the bluish purple of blueberries. These fruits and vegetables tend to be rich sources of anthocyanins, a group of phytonutrients shown to promote brain health.

How do anthocyanins work? Anthocyanins have powerful antioxidant and anti-inflammatory actions. In the brain (and throughout the body), antioxidants help protect cells from the so-called "free radicals" that result from normal cellular metabolism. When the brain is unable to neutralize these unstable biochemical byproducts, a state of oxidative stress occurs that can damage and destroy healthy brain cells. A well-nourished brain, by contrast, is primed to neutralize these destructive free radicals thanks, in large part, to a diet rich in antioxidants, including anthocyanins.

Anthocyanins help combat oxidative stress in two important ways. First, they work by interacting directly with unstable free radicals to trap and neutralize them. Next, anthocyanins work by supporting the cell's own ability to produce antioxidants. Think of it as a dual-action antioxidant defense your child needs to support brain health and optimal cognitive function.

Let's take a deeper dive into why encouraging your child to eat more anthocyanin-rich purple foods can help them stay at the top of their mental game.

Parent Pearl

Soup for the soul. When the weather starts to cool down, I find the best way to warm up my family is with a bowl of soup. A simmering kettle of fresh vegetable soup coupled with a crusty whole grain roll makes for a wonderful and nourishing dinner.

The "Brainberry"

One of the stars of the purple group is the blueberry, which is both kid-friendly and brimming with anthocyanins. This tiny berry packs some mighty brain benefits earning it the prestigious nickname "brainberry."

Over 20 years ago, researchers discovered laboratory rats fed the equivalent of 1 cup of blueberries each day for two months improved their short-term memory. Remembering a maze that ends in a cheesy reward is a good thing for a laboratory rat, but what about kids? Does feeding young kids a serving of blueberries affect their mental sharpness? Turns out, it does.

In one systematic review,[3] Dr Nikolaj Travica at Swinburne University of Technology in Australia and colleagues evaluated 12 well-controlled clinical trials investigating blueberry intake and cognitive performance in kids, teens and adults. Five trials focused on kids ranging from 7 to 10 years of age, and the results were compelling. Eating a test meal with blueberries (compared to one without) significantly improved memory, recall and other mental functions in as little as 2 hours. These brainy benefits were seen with a 30-gram serving of freeze-dried wild blueberries (about 3 tablespoons) and with a 200-gram serving of fresh blueberries (about 1⅓ cups). As you may have guessed, both are rich sources of anthocyanins.

How does your child's intake of fruits and vegetables in the purple group rate? Take our **Purple Power Assessment** find out.

Purple Power Assessment

Check (☑) the box for each food below that your child eats. Enter the total number of foods at the bottom. Read on to learn how your child's diet rates.

- ❑ Acai berries
- ❑ Asparagus (purple)
- ❑ Basil (purple)
- ❑ Beets
- ❑ Bell peppers (purple)
- ❑ Blackberries
- ❑ Blueberries
- ❑ Boysenberries
- ❑ Cabbage (red)
- ❑ Other:_____

- ❑ Carrots (purple)
- ❑ Currants (black)
- ❑ Dates
- ❑ Eggplant
- ❑ Elderberries
- ❑ Figs (purple)
- ❑ Grapes (Concord)
- ❑ Huckleberries
- ❑ Kale (purple)

- ❑ Kohlrabi (purple)
- ❑ Olallieberries
- ❑ Plum
- ❑ Potato (purple)
- ❑ Pluots
- ❑ Prunes
- ❑ Raisins
- ❑ Rhubarb

Enter the total number here.

How Did Your Child Do?

If your child currently consumes more than 10 different purple fruits and vegetables, you both deserve a big pat on the back. Bravo! If not, consider adding one or two more purple fruits or vegetables to your family's diet this month. Make it a fun adventure as you shop for these purple beauties at your local grocery or farmers market. Don't forget the frozen section, where out-of-season produce such as blueberries, can be found year round.

The Red Group

The bright red color of tomatoes comes from lycopene, a plant compound that's also responsible for the vibrant color of other red fruits and vegetables like watermelon, mango, papaya and guava. It's one you'll want to focus on because lycopene is a powerful antioxidant that promotes heart and circulatory health.[4]

That's good news for an active brain because healthy circulation means blood can carry nutrients to your child's brain and whisk away metabolic waste with ease. Plus, some red fruits and vegetables also contain anthocyanins. As you just learned, anthocyanins and their antioxidant and anti-inflammatory properties are more commonly found in the purple color group. Nonetheless, it's a nice bonus to see in the red group because it all adds up to serious support for a well-nourished brain, one that can function at peak performance.

So, how does your child's intake of red fruits and vegetables rate? Take our **Red Rocks Assessment** to find out.

Parent Pearl

Consider adding pomegranate seeds to your child's diet. We do this at home and they are a true crowd pleaser. Just make sure you have plenty of napkins!

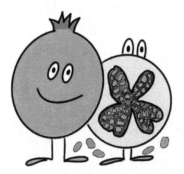

Red Rocks Assessment

Check (☑) the box for each food below that your child eats. Enter the total number of foods at the bottom. Read on to learn how your child's diet rates.

- ❑ Apple (red)[†]
- ❑ Bell pepper (red)
- ❑ Cabbage (red)[†]
- ❑ Cherries[†]
- ❑ Chokeberries[†]
- ❑ Cranberries[†]
- ❑ Currants (red)[†]
- ❑ Grapefruit (pink, red)[*]
- ❑ Grapes (red)[†]
- ❑ Other:_____

- ❑ Kidney beans (red)[†]
- ❑ Lettuce (red)[†]
- ❑ Mango
- ❑ Onion (red)[†]
- ❑ Papaya (pink)[*]
- ❑ Pomegranate[†]
- ❑ Potatoes (red)[†]
- ❑ Radicchio
- ❑ Radishes (red)[†]

- ❑ Raspberries (red)[†]
- ❑ Rhubarb[†]
- ❑ Strawberries[†]
- ❑ Tomato (including tomato paste, ketchup and spaghetti sauce)[*]
- ❑ Watermelon[*]

* rich in lycopene[5]
† rich in anthocyanins[6,7]

❑ Enter the total number here.

How Did Your Child Do?

If your child currently consumes more than 10 different red fruits and vegetables, excellent! If not, consider adding one or two more to your family's diet this month. In this case, even ketchup and spaghetti sauce count because they're loaded with lycopene.

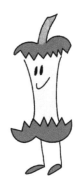

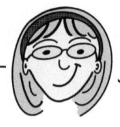

Did You Know?

You absorb more lycopene when you cook tomatoes with olive oil and fresh, diced onions. This tasty discovery is published in the October 2019 issue of *Food Chemistry*.

The researchers found that cooking tomatoes in olive oil alone has little effect on its lycopene content. But, when pureed onions were added to the mix, the tomato lycopene converted to a form more readily absorbed by the body.

Turns out, pureeing onions activates enzymes that release sulfur-containing compounds that, in turn, act as a catalyst to improve the bioavailability of lycopene. Blanched onions won't work (blanching kills the enzymes needed to make the sulfur compounds). The onions need to be fresh, which is one more reason to buy your produce, preferably organic, at your local farmer's market.[8]

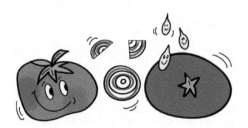

The Orange-Yellow Group

Fruits and vegetables in the orange-yellow group tend to be rich in phytonutrients known as carotenoids such as alpha-carotene, beta-carotene, beta-cryptoxanthin, lutein and zeaxanthin. Fruits and vegetables with these brain-protecting antioxidants are also being studied for their potential benefits for heart and immune health and healthy vision.

As you learned in the previous chapter, lutein is especially important for healthy vision. This plant pigment is why foods like corn and egg yolks are yellow, but it's also found in leafy green vegetables like spinach and kale (it's hiding under the green of chlorophyll.) Once consumed, lutein travels to the macula, the area of the eye responsible for sharp vision, where it absorbs harmful high-energy blue light (the same light emitted by typical video display screens).[9]

If you think lutein sounds like a nutritional shield for your eyes, you're right. Add regular blinking breaks, and you just may banish tired, sore eyes for good.

How does your child's intake of these orange-yellow beauties rate? Take our **Outrageous Orange-Yellow Assessment** on page 69 to find out.

Parent Pearl

Show them they're a star! My kids love the exotic carambola fruit. To make this yellow-orange fruit extra special, I slice crosswise and serve up the natural star-shaped slices. It's a delicious way to boost nutrition.

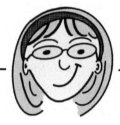

Did You Know?

The Have a Plant® Movement is an educational program offered by the non-profit Produce for Better Health Foundation. It offers a wealth of expert advice on fruits and veggies. You'll find a library of fun facts, practical planning, shopping and cooking tips and more for hundreds of fruits and vegetables—all focused on inspiring kids (and adults) to eat more fruits and veggies. Learn more at https://fruitsandveggies.org.

Outrageous Orange-Yellow Assessment

Check (☑) the box for each food below that your child eats. Enter the total number of foods at the bottom. Read on to learn how your child's diet rates.

- ❏ Apple (yellow)
- ❏ Apricots*
- ❏ Pears (Asian)
- ❏ Bell pepper (yellow, orange)*
- ❏ Cantaloupe*
- ❏ Cape gooseberries
- ❏ Carambola (star fruit)*
- ❏ Carrot*
- ❏ Cherries (yellow)
- ❏ Corn*

- ❏ Dill
- ❏ Kumquats
- ❏ Lemon
- ❏ Mango*
- ❏ Melon (casaba, Crenshaw, Persian)
- ❏ Mint
- ❏ Nectarine
- ❏ Orange
- ❏ Papaya

- ❏ Parsley
- ❏ Passion fruit
- ❏ Peach
- ❏ Pear (golden)
- ❏ Persimmon*
- ❏ Pineapple
- ❏ Plantain
- ❏ Potato (yellow)
- ❏ Pumpkin*
- ❏ Quince
- ❏ Tangelo
- ❏ Tangerine*

- ❏ Rutabaga
- ❏ Summer squash (yellow)*
- ❏ Sweet potato*
- ❏ Winter squash (acorn, banana, butternut, spaghetti)*
- ❏ Yam*

Other:_____

* rich in alpha-carotene, beta-carotene, lutein or zeaxanthin[5]

Enter the total number here.

How Did Your Child Do?

If your child's diet includes 15 or more fruits and vegetables in the orange-yellow color group, great job! If it includes between eight and 10 of these carotenoid-rich beauties, it's still a job well done. For more variety, consider adding another orange-yellow fruit or veggie to your child's diet each week until they're enjoying enough of these protective foods. If fewer than eight are showing up in your child's diet, it's time to focus. Pull out the cookbooks, and use your creative juices. You may be surprised at the results.

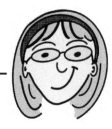

Did You Know?

The phytonutrients in different colored fruits and veggies deliver distinct health benefits. Ask your child to study a fruit or vegetable and describe what they see—the star on a blueberry or the golden-red splotches on a peach. Remind your child that each color works in its own special way to protect both body and brain.[10]

The Green Group

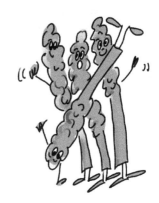

Fruits and vegetables in the green group contain a wide variety of beneficial phytonutrients. For example, vegetables in the cruciferous family such as broccoli, kale, collard greens and bok choy are natural sources of sulforaphane, isothiocyanates and other phytonutrients with tongue-twister names. These plant powerhouses rev up the liver's production of enzymes that help keep cells throughout the body healthy.

Plus, as you learned earlier, spinach, kale and other leafy green vegetables are also good sources of lutein, the yellow phytonutrient. The green of chlorophyll hides this antioxidant powerhouse, but it's there.

How does your child's intake of fruits and vegetables in the green group rate? Take our **Go Green Assessment** on the next page to find out.

Go Green Assessment

Check (☑) the box for each food below that your child eats. Enter the total number of foods at the bottom. Read on to learn how your child's diet rates.

- ❑ Apple (green)
- ❑ Artichoke
- ❑ Arugula
- ❑ Asparagus
- ❑ Avocado
- ❑ Beet greens
- ❑ Bell pepper (green)
- ❑ Bok choy*
- ❑ Broccoli*
- ❑ Broccoflower*
- ❑ Brussels sprouts*
- ❑ Cabbage (green)
- ❑ Cactus
- ❑ Celery
- ❑ Other:_____

- ❑ Collard greens*
- ❑ Cucumber
- ❑ Dandelion greens
- ❑ Fennel
- ❑ Grapes (green)
- ❑ Green beans
- ❑ Honeydew melon
- ❑ Kale*
- ❑ Kiwi
- ❑ Leek
- ❑ Lettuce (butter, iceberg, romaine, etc.)
- ❑ Lima beans
- ❑ Lime

- ❑ Mustard greens*
- ❑ Okra
- ❑ Onion (green)
- ❑ Pear (green)
- ❑ Peas (green, snow, sugar snap)
- ❑ Spinach
- ❑ Swiss chard*
- ❑ Turnip greens
- ❑ Watercress
- ❑ Wax beans
- ❑ Zucchini

* rich in isothiocyanates or indoles

❑ Enter the total number here.

How Did Your Child Do?

If your child's diet includes 20 or more fruits and vegetables in the green color group, great job! If it includes between eight and 19 greens, that's still impressive. But, if your child squeaked out fewer than eight, it's time to revisit the list of foods to select more. The good news is, with so many kid-friendly greens to choose from, it's relatively easy to add a few more to your child's diet.

The White & Brown Group

White and brown fruits and vegetables may lack vibrant colors, but that doesn't mean they don't pack a nutritious punch. For example, vegetables in the allium family like onions, garlic, chives, leeks and shallots contain allicin. This phytonutrient exerts powerful antioxidant activity that promotes circulatory health and supports the function of the immune system. Onions and garlic, as well as apples, are also sources of another naturally occurring phytonutrient called quercetin, which works to promote a healthy inflammatory response.

How does your child's intake of fruits and vegetables in this color group rate? Take our **Wonderful White & Brown Assessment** on page 75 to find out.

Parent Pearl

For an exotic treat, I serve cherimoya. With white flesh and black almond-shaped seeds, this fruit has a texture like custard but tastes like a blend of banana, pineapple and papaya. And, it's a good source of vitamin C and fiber. The kids love it, especially when chilled.

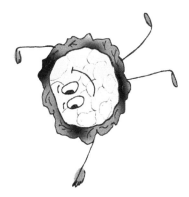

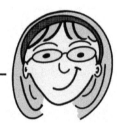

Did You Know?

You can encourage your child to be an artist when it comes to selecting fruits and vegetables. Think of it as painting a rainbow on the plate using as many of the color groups as possible—red, orange-yellow, green, purple and white-brown. The more colors, the better for your child's diet. As a general rule, have your child include at least three natural colors on their plate at meal times. Make it a game; see who can design the most colorful plate.

Wonderful White & Brown Assessment

Check (☑) the box for each food below that your child eats. Enter the total number of foods at the bottom. Read on to see how your child's diet rates.

- ❑ Banana
- ❑ Belgian endive
- ❑ Black beans
- ❑ Cauliflower
- ❑ Celery root
- ❑ Chayote squash
- ❑ Cherimoya
- ❑ Other:_____

- ❑ Chestnuts
- ❑ Chives*
- ❑ Coconut
- ❑ Dates
- ❑ Garlic*
- ❑ Ginger
- ❑ Jicama

- ❑ Kohlrabi
- ❑ Leek*
- ❑ Morels
- ❑ Mushrooms
- ❑ Onion (white)*
- ❑ Parsnip
- ❑ Pinto beans

- ❑ Potato (russet)
- ❑ Radishes
- ❑ Rutabaga
- ❑ Shallots*
- ❑ Turnip

* rich in allicin

❑ Enter the total number here.

How Did Your Child Do?

If your child's diet includes 12 or more fruits and vegetables in the white and brown color group, you're really a superstar. (It can be tough to get a wide variety in this group). If it includes between eight and 11 whites and browns, give yourself a pat on the back, but don't forget to work on boosting the variety.

If your child's diet has fewer than seven foods in this color group, this is where extra focus will pay off. Consider adding a new food into your child's diet this week. Continue each week until your child is enjoying at least eight different fruits and veggies in this color group on a regular basis.

Active Brains Benefit from Variety

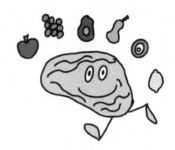

When it comes to choosing fruits and veggies to include in your child's diet, the more variety, the better. So, top on your list of brain-boosting goals should be including a wide range of richly colored fruits and vegetables on your child's plate every day. What's more, focusing on including a variety of colorful fruits and vegetables in your child's diet will help ensure their intake is optimal for overall health and wellbeing.

Unfortunately, many children fail to consume the daily recommended intake of fruits and vegetables. It's a dismal trend that extends across all age groups, according to the Dietary Guidelines for Americans (2020–2025).[11] From pre-K to elementary school and beyond, kids consistently fall short of the recommended intakes for fruits and vegetables.

But, there's good news: It only takes a few cups a day for your child to nourish their body and brain. In other words, it's a habit that's doable, you just need to start.

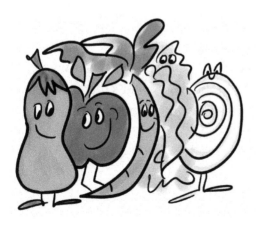

How Much Should Your Child Eat?

Experts recommend children eat at least 3 to 5 servings of fruits and vegetables every day, depending on their age, sex and activity level. The chart below provides a quick reference guide. However, when it comes to consuming fruits and vegetables, the general rule is: The more, the better, especially for vegetables.

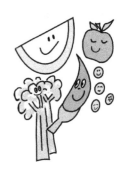

Recommended Daily Servings of Fruit and Vegetable for Children*		
Grade (Age)	**Fruits**	**Vegetables**
Kindergarten (5 to 6 years)	1½	1½ to 2
First Grade (6 to 7 years)	1½	1½ to 2
Second Grade (7 to 8 years)	1½	1½ to 2
Third Grade (8 to 9 years)	1½	1½ to 2
Fourth Grade (9 to 10 years)	1½ to 2	2 to 2½ (girls) 2 to 3 (boys)
Fifth Grade (10 to 11 years)	1½ to 2	2 to 2½ (girls) 2 to 3 (boys)
Sixth Grade (11 to 12 years)	1½ to 2 cups	2 to 2½ cups (girls) 2 to 3 cups (boys)
* For a moderately active child (30-60 minutes of activity per day). Children who are more or less physically active may require more or less, respectively, to meet their needs. Source: Dietary Guidelines for Americans (2020-2025).		

For more information about serving sizes, see **Sample Serving Sizes for Each Food Group** on page 288.

Six Easy Steps to More Fruits & Veggies

1 **Keep fruits and vegetables visible.** Fill a fruit bowl and put it in an easily accessible spot in your kitchen, or place a tray full of ready-to-munch raw vegetables in the refrigerator at your child's eye level. (For more ideas about keeping healthy foods within arm's reach, see **Stocking Your Fridge, Freezer & Pantry** on page 279.)

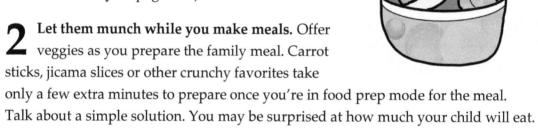

2 **Let them munch while you make meals.** Offer veggies as you prepare the family meal. Carrot sticks, jicama slices or other crunchy favorites take only a few extra minutes to prepare once you're in food prep mode for the meal. Talk about a simple solution. You may be surprised at how much your child will eat.

3 **Slip in extra helpings of veggies and fruits.** Consider adding finely chopped carrots, eggplant, broccoli, cauliflower or other veggies to marinara sauce, soups, stews and chili. Try stuffing a pita pocket with veggie chunks or offering a fruit salad or smoothie as a snack or dessert.

4 **Try roasting vegetables for a deep, rich flavor.** Drizzle veggies with a little olive oil and roast in an oven set to 425 degrees Fahrenheit or on the grill until tender. Try carrots, asparagus, butternut squash, eggplant, broccoli or just about any vegetable that you like.

5 **Pack and go.** Toss snap peas, soybeans, carrots, jicama, baby tomatoes or other pieces of raw vegetables in a plastic bag for your child to munch on when away from home.

6 **Let them choose.** When grocery shopping, allow your child to select a fruit or vegetable that he or she wants to eat.

Organic: Is It Really Better?

Some of the most common questions about organically grown fruits and vegetables are whether they're more nutritious, tastier and safer than conventionally grown varieties. Read on to learn what researchers know (and don't know):

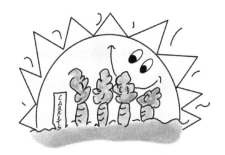

Are organic foods more nutritious?

The jury is still out. There are only a few well-controlled studies comparing the nutrient content of organic and conventionally grown fruits and vegetables. In general, these studies fail to show a significant difference in the amounts of micronutrients such as vitamins, minerals and trace elements. However, there appears to be a slight trend toward higher vitamin C content in organically grown leafy vegetables and potatoes.

Are organic foods tastier?

Some folks say that organic foods taste much better than conventionally grown foods. Others say there's no difference. Since taste is a subjective matter, only you would be the best judge. Whether you decide to buy foods that are grown organically or conventionally, choosing the freshest foods available is likely to have the biggest impact on taste. If possible, choose locally grown foods as these tend to be the freshest.

Are organic foods safer?

In a word, yes. A growing body of academic research conducted in the United States indicates that switching to an organic diet can help dramatically reduce a child's body burden of pesticides. And, it doesn't take long. In one study,[12] Dr. Chensheng Lu and colleagues at Emory University found the level of pesticides in children's urine plummeted to undetectable levels after only five days on an organic diet. In another study,[13] Dr. Asa Bradman and colleagues at U.C. Berkeley found an organic diet significantly reduced pesticide residue levels in children's urine after only seven days. In yet another study,[14] Dr. Carly Hyland, also at U.C. Berkeley, and colleagues found urinary levels of 13 pesticide residues from commonly used pesticides in conventional agriculture significantly dropped after only six days on the organic diet. If you're sensing a theme here, you're right. If you want to reduce your child's pesticide load, going organic works, and it works fast.

Should you be worried?

Researchers continue to debate the health risks of pesticide exposure for children, including its effect on attention, behavior and learning. But, one thing is certain: Pesticides are neurotoxins. They kill bugs by paralyzing or over-exciting their nervous systems. So, it makes sense that reducing your child's exposure to these same toxins can go a long way to protecting their brain. Choosing organic foods whenever possible can help.

An Easy Way to Avoid Pesticides

While the amounts of pesticide residue in fruits and vegetables varies, you can keep your child's exposure to a minimum by using the Shopper's Guide to Pesticides in Produce™ published annually by the Environmental Working Group (EWG).[15]

To come up with its rankings, the EWG examines the results of thousands of tests for pesticides on produce performed by the USDA and the U.S. Food and Drug Administration. The 12 fruits and vegetables that consistently have the highest levels of pesticides are dubbed the "Dirty Dozen." Strawberries top the list published in 2023. Conversely, the "Clean 15" list represents those fruits and vegetables with the lowest pesticide residue.

If your child's favorites are among the Dirty Dozen, buy organic whenever possible. If you don't see your child's favorites, visit www.ewg.org. Here you'll find full lists as well as updated lists as they become available each year.

The "Dirty Dozen"
(Highest in Pesticide Residue)

1. Strawberries
2. Spinach
3. Kale, Collard & Mustard Greens
4. Peaches
5. Pears
6. Nectarines
7. Apples
8. Grapes
9. Bell & Hot Peppers
10. Cherries
11. Blueberries
12. Green Beans

The "Clean 15"
(Lowest in Pesticide Residue)

1. Avocado
2. Sweet Corn*
3. Pineapple
4. Onion
5. Papaya*
6. Sweet Peas (frozen)
7. Asparagus
8. Honeydew Melon
9. Kiwi
10. Cabbage
11. Mushrooms
12. Mango
13. Sweet Potatoes
14. Watermelon
15. Carrots

*Some sweet corn (as well as papayas and summer squash) sold in the United States is produced from genetically modified seeds. To avoid or limit your intake of genetically modified products, buy organic.
Source: Environmental Working Group's 2023 Shoppers Guide to Pesticides in Produce™.

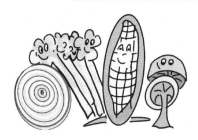

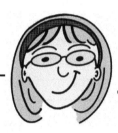

Did You Know?

You can find a registered dietitian in your area who specializes in child nutrition by asking your pediatrician for a recommendation. You can also visit the Academy of Nutrition and Dietetics website (www.eatright.org). Click on the "Find a Nutrition Expert" tab, and you'll be able to search a national database of credentialed and licensed nutrition professionals by location, telemedicine services, specialty, languages, and insurance options.

Healthy Choices for Every Budget

In general, organic foods are more expensive than conventional foods. But, you don't need to choose 100% organic fruits and vegetables to get protective benefits. With four simple food shopping and preparation tips, you can make healthier choices yet remain budget-conscious. Here's how:

1 **Review the "Dirty Dozen" list.** If your child's favorites are on the list, focus on buying those foods organically grown.

2 **Wash and peel.** Wash fruits and vegetables thoroughly. If you're concerned about pesticides, peel your fruits and vegetables and trim outer leaves of leafy vegetables.

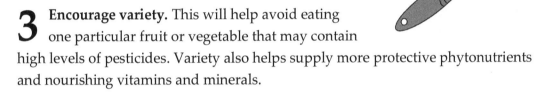

3 **Encourage variety.** This will help avoid eating one particular fruit or vegetable that may contain high levels of pesticides. Variety also helps supply more protective phytonutrients and nourishing vitamins and minerals.

4 **Look at the big picture.** If your child's diet is full of processed and fast foods, it's best to begin by making more general lifestyle changes such as having them eat more fruits and vegetables, legumes and whole grains—whether they are organic or not—and eat less processed, refined and fast foods. When this becomes a regular habit, then consider exploring organic options. Remember, it's not a race to good nutrition. It's a step-by-step, one-day-at-a-time process that leads to a lifetime of healthful eating. Your child will get there.

This Month's Smart Goal

I will add one serving of fruits or vegetables each week until my child meets the recommended intake (at least 3 to 5 servings daily based on age).

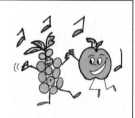

This Month's Extra Credit

I will serve a fruit or veggie in each color group (purple, red, orange-yellow, green and white-brown) every day.*

*While every day is preferable, start with where you are and slowly build up.

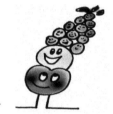

To monitor your daily progress toward your goals, use the **My Smart Tracker** forms in **Chapter 14: Go for the Goal.**

Part 3

Winter Season

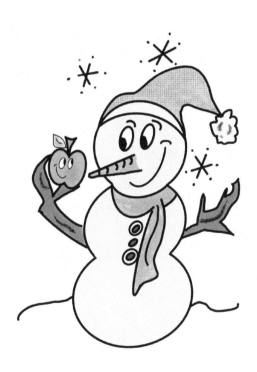

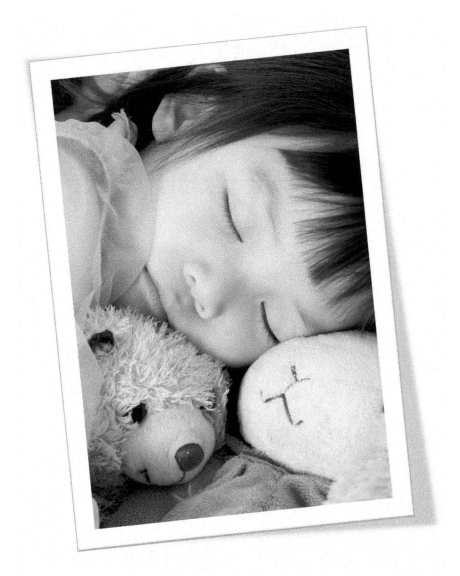

A good laugh and a long sleep are
the best cures in the doctor's book.
                    — Irish Proverb

Chapter 5

December – Sleep, De-Stress & Learn

Sleep and memory experts have long known getting enough zzz's influences how a child performs in the classroom. It's easy to understand when you know the two ways that sleep powers your child's mental abilities. First, adequate sleep is essential for overall good mental performance. Second, sleep is a key player in how a child's brain consolidates, refines and converts new skills and learning into lasting memories. This process of memory consolidation is critical for a child to form long-term memories so they can navigate their world (both physical and abstract).[1]

So, no matter what's on your child's daily To-Do list—studying for a spelling test, preparing for a piano recital or perfecting the latest skateboard move—make sure their day of learning is followed by a full night of restorative sleep.

The Power of REM Sleep

Just what kind of sleep triggers memory benefits? It's REM sleep, the so-called deep sleep characterized by rapid eye movements. Throughout the night, we tend to alternate between

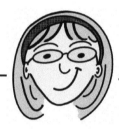

Did You Know?

Sleep experts at the National Sleep Foundation agree that screen time too close to bedtime not only makes it difficult for kids to fall asleep, it can also rob them of the much-needed total hours of sleep. Aim to turn off the television and other electronics at least one hour before bedtime. (You may need to start with 10 or 20 minutes and build up from there.) For more tips on promoting a happy slumber for kids and adults alike, visit www.sleepfoundation.org.

memory-boosting REM sleep and non-REM sleep every 90 minutes or so. That means, with a good night's sleep, your child's brain has the opportunity to actively process the day's events, strengthen memories and possibly gain new insights about learned activities. Read on for nine ways you can help your child get enough memory-enhancing REM sleep.

9 Ways to Promote Memory-Enhancing Sleep

1 **Get enough hours of sleep.** The amount of sleep your child needs each night depends on their age. According to the U.S. National Sleep Foundation (www.sleepfoundation.org), current recommendations range from 10 to 13 hours for preschool children, 9 to 11 hours for older children, and 8 to 10 hours for teens.

2 **Stick to a routine.** Going to bed and waking up at the same time, even during the weekends, supports your child's natural 24-hour circadian rhythm and helps shape a solid sleep-promoting schedule. Avoid the temptation to make up for lost sleep by sleeping more on the weekend. It doesn't work that way. Worse, it makes it harder to wake up during the week.

3 **Keep the bedroom cool, dark and quiet.** Make sure your child's bedroom has the basics for a comfortable night's sleep: cool temperature, dark room and minimal noise.

4 **Keep electronics and LED lights out of the bedroom.** Electronics and artificial lights emit blue light. Light in this wavelength can trick the brain into thinking it's daytime, which can lead to sleep problems.

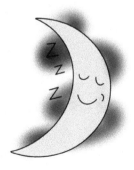

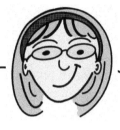

Did You Know?

Sleep problems are common in children and can take a serious toll on their cognitive, emotional and behavioral development.[2] This lack of adequate sleep causes kids to be more than just tired, they also have a harder time paying attention and thinking clearly, not to mention controlling their impulses and emotions. In fact, a sleep-deprived child can exhibit all the signs of Attention-Deficit /Hyperactivity Disorder (ADHD). In other words, being tired, distracted and cranky is a serious barrier to effective learning. Yet, the fix could be as simple as making sure your child gets an extra 30 minutes of nightly sleep. It's well worth the effort given the critical role sleep plays in a child's cognitive development and school performance.[3]

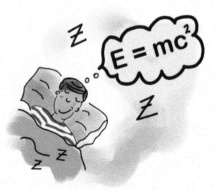

5 **Limit fluids after dinner.** This will help reduce the need to wake up for those midnight trips to the bathroom. Should nature call, consider using a night-light to help guide the way.

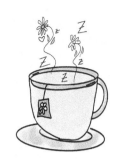

6 **Avoid caffeine-containing drinks.** It's best for kids to avoid caffeine-containing foods and beverages because the stimulating effects of caffeine can last for several hours after that last sip. So, when it comes to helping your little one drift off into sound slumber, the less caffeine consumed, especially after 3 p.m., the better.

7 **Set phone to wind down mode.** Most smart phones have a wind down mode that helps reduce distraction before bedtime so your child can relax and fall asleep.

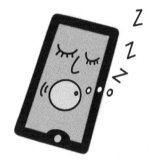

8 **Soothing slumber.** Consider offering your child a soothing cup of chamomile tea. This calming herb has a history of traditional use that hails back to the ancient Egyptians, Greeks and Romans. It remains popular today because, well, it works.

9 **Rise and shine, naturally.** If your child has trouble getting up in the morning, check out some of the sunrise alarm clocks designed to help your child wake up naturally by mimicking the dawn's early light.

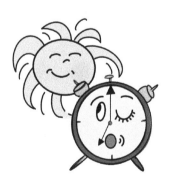

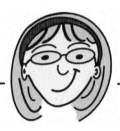

Did You Know?

Kids have a natural preference for how they learn whether it's by seeing, hearing or doing. Tap into your child's preferred method, and learning will seem almost effortless.

Reduce Emotional Stress, Boost Mental Function

If you feel like your kids are under a lot of emotional stress these days, you're not wrong. Many parents are seeing the telltale signs of a stressed-out kid like unusual outbursts, frustration and irritability, not to mention trouble sleeping. The good news is you can make stress work for your child. It's all about balance. Read on for a few simple ways to help your child destress so they can feel calm, cool and collected.

Think balance

Kids need some stress to get moving and be productive, but too much can put them on overload. It's like the strings on a violin. Too loose, and the music moans and groans. Too tight, and the music shrieks. Only the right amount of tension produces beautiful music. It's the same with stress. When your child is able to balance their stress level, they're better prepared to excel in school and in life. For this reason, it's important for them to do something every day to balance stress.

Make time to reflect

Doing too much without enough rest can leave your child feeling physically drained, unable to focus and just plain overwhelmed. There's one way to banish this pressure-cooker feeling, and it's free, easy and only takes a few minutes. Ask your child take a few minutes to stop what they're doing and just look at the world around them. Listen to the sounds, take in the sights and be present in the moment.

It may seem counter-intuitive, but taking time each day to slow down, even just a little bit, can help bring calm to the rest of your child's day, help them be more productive and ultimately be their best self. Really, it's

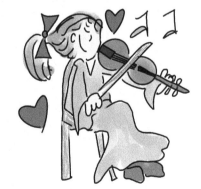

that simple. Yet, many parents are unaware of the huge benefits this daily habit has to help a child destress.

Here's how to help your child get started. First, set aside 15 minutes each day to just observe the world. If this feels like forever, that's OK. Start with a shorter length of time, say 5 minutes, and build up from there.

Next, ask your child to breathe deeply as they take in the surrounding sights and sounds that fill the air, inhaling slowly through their nose and exhaling through their mouth. (They can place their hand on their belly to make sure it expands when they inhale, so they know they're breathing deeply.)

Have them take it all in, quietly and with intention. Make this a daily habit, and your child will likely feel calmer throughout the day. Even better, this mindful practice can help them feel more resilient. In other words, it's a simple habit with serious benefits for your child's emotional wellbeing.

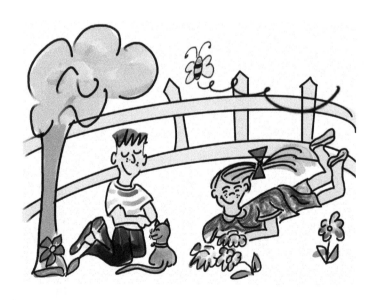

Five Stress-Busters for Better Balance

To help your child feel calm and focused throughout the day, consider putting one or more of the stress-busters below into practice right now:

1 **Balance school, play, family and friendships.** Like a violin with four strings, your child needs all four areas of their life in balance so their mind, body and spirit can flourish.

2 **Use a daily planner.** Writing down all your child's activities on a master schedule (including homework assignments) can help you better manage your time and keep your child calm and focused.

3 **Break big projects into smaller chunks.** If a project feels overwhelming to your child, encourage them to break it down into smaller tasks and chip away at it on a regular basis. In this way, they're more likely to complete the project on time without losing sleep or feeling too stressed.

4 **Fill the air with a favorite scent.** How about lavender, citrus or coconut? Your child (and you) will breathe deeper, which helps lower heart rate and blood pressure.

5 **Fill tummies with stress-busting nutrients.** While the oxidative stress you learned about in the previous chapter is less apparent than the feelings of emotional stress (rapid heart rate, tense muscles and rapid breathing), it's just as harmful. As you learned, eating a variety of antioxidant-rich plant foods can help shield growing brains (and bodies) from the harmful effects of this toxic form of stress. It's one more reason to fill your child's plate with fruits and vegetables, nuts, herbs and spices.

Parent Pearl

I fill an extra salt shaker with cinnamon and keep it handy. It's an easy way to help my kids sprinkle this antioxidant-rich spice on foods.

For a Happier Day, Move More

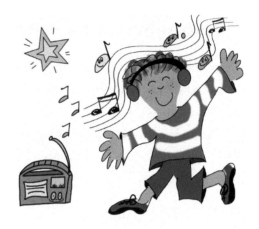

You can have a happier child right now (ok within an hour), you just need to get them moving. In general, kids who are more physically active are happier over the long run.

But there's also an immediate benefit. In one study,[4] researchers in the Netherlands followed more than 1,480 kids between the ages of 8 to 17 years who were given a so-called "wearable lab" that included a wrist fitness tracker and a smartphone. The fitness tracker was used to count steps and track physical activity, minute by minute, for a maximum of five days. The smartphone allowed the children to reply to randomly timed requests to rate how happy they were at that specific moment.

Turns out, the number of steps accumulated in a given hour predicted happiness in the next hour. In fact, adding as few as 1,000 steps to the typical daily activity level was enough to shift into happier state of mind for that day (more was better).

For physical health, experts recommend kids get 60 minutes or more of moderate to vigorous activity every day.[5] Adding a few more steps could also mean a happier day.

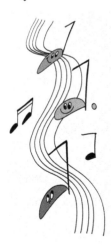

If you need inspiration to get your child moving, consider adding a little music to their routine. After all, research shows music makes exercise more enjoyable, improves performance, helps reduce perceived exertion and improves oxygen consumption. In other words, music helps delay fatigue so your child feels like staying active longer.[6] A definite win, win.

This Month's Smart Goal

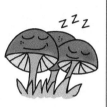

I will enforce a regular bedtime hour to help my child get enough memory-enhancing REM sleep at least five times per week.

This Month's Extra Credit

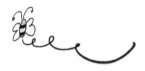

I will have my child take at least 5 minutes a day to stop, listen and learn (and really "bee" present in the moment).

To monitor your daily progress toward your goals, use the **My Smart Tracker** forms in **Chapter 14: Go for the Goal.**

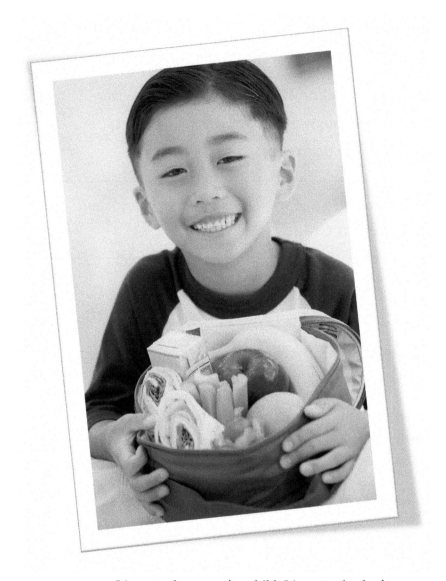

Listen to the mustn'ts, child. Listen to the don'ts.
Listen to the shouldn'ts, the impossibles, the won'ts.
Listen to the never haves, then listen close to me ...
Anything can happen, child. Anything can be.
— Shel Silverstein

Chapter 6

January – Pack a Power Lunch

Can you believe it? The school year is almost half over. As time marches on, your beginning-of-the-year exuberance about packing your child's school lunch may be fizzling out. If you need a little inspiration to jazz up your menus, this chapter is for you. You'll learn new ways to revitalize the mid-day meal with both brain-building nutrition and kid-friendly flavor to satisfy both you and your child.

While a healthy breakfast gets your kid's engine revving for their morning classes, lunch provides critical fuel for the home stretch. In fact, packing a power lunch is essential for your child to maintain focus and attention during those afternoon classes. It's easier than you may think when you focus on the nutrition essentials for energy, alertness and memory.

Carbs for Energy

Foods rich in carbohydrates provide the fuel to keep your child active throughout the school day. There are two types of carbohydrates: simple and complex.

Simple Carbohydrates

Simple carbohydrates provide quick energy. Chemically speaking, simple carbohydrates are made up of only one or two building blocks of sugar. Because of their simple structure, it doesn't take long for them to break down, be absorbed and used for energy in your child's body. This is the reason they are often referred to as "quick energy."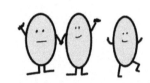
Examples include sucrose (white table sugar), fructose (fruit sugar) and lactose (milk sugar). Each of these simple sugars end with the letters "ose," which simply means sugar.

Complex Carbohydrates

Complex carbohydrates are made up of chains of simple sugars and provide long-sustaining energy. Before complex carbohydrates can be absorbed and utilized in your child's body, they must first be broken down.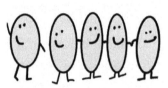

It all starts with amylase, a digestive enzyme that helps slowly break down a complex carbohydrate, releasing one sugar molecule at a time. Once a sugar molecule is broken off, it can be absorbed and used by the body for energy. Because this process takes time, it results in the sustained increase in energy that complex carbohydrates provide. Foods rich in complex carbohydrates include bread, starchy vegetables, cereals and other grain products.

Your Best Bets

The best carbohydrates are those that come from unrefined sources. Think fruits in terms of simple carbohydrates. Think beans, legumes, starchy vegetables and 100% whole grains in terms of complex carbohydrates. These choices are richer in vitamins, minerals, fiber and phytonutrients.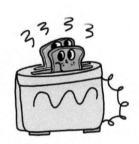

Think of a Pearl

You can help your child understand the concept of simple and complex carbohydrates by using a pearl analogy.

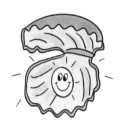

Ask your child to think of a pearl. It's like the simple carbohydrates (simple sugars) found in sodas, sweets, fruits, milk and similar foods. Let your child know that this type of carbohydrate melts in the mouth and is quickly absorbed by the body. It provides a short burst of energy, but can be followed by fatigue.

Now, ask your child to imagine a strand of pearls. It's like a complex carbohydrate. When you string simple sugars together—like a strand of pearls—they become a complex carbohydrate. In order for the body to use complex carbohydrates for energy, it must break off one simple sugar at a time. It's like taking one pearl at a time off a pearl necklace. Since this is a slow process, energy is released slowly over time to deliver long-lasting energy. This is one of the key reasons why complex carbohydrates are the preferred fuel for your child's body.

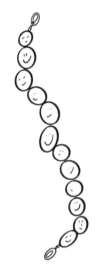

Quality Counts

You can take this analogy one step further. Just as fake pearls are lower quality than their genuine counterparts, simple sugars from refined sources are lower quality, providing empty calories and little, if any, nutritional value. By contrast, the unrefined simple sugars found in fruits and many vegetables are like a genuine pearl with their high-quality nutrition bundled with vitamins, minerals and phytonutrients.

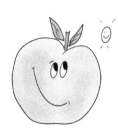

Similarly, unrefined complex carbohydrates found in 100% whole grains (as opposed to refined varieties such as white bread, white rice and white flour) are also like a genuine pearl necklace. These too are high-quality sources bundled with vitamins, minerals and dietary fiber. And, just like a genuine pearl necklace looks better over time, unrefined carbohydrates—whether simple or complex—are better for the body over time.

Protein to Stay Alert

Protein is important for strong muscles, but did you know that it also helps keep your child alert? This is especially important in the mid-afternoon when kids tend to start dragging, and their attention begins to wander.

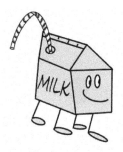

Protein-rich Brain Foods

- Milk, yogurt, cheese, egg whites
- Lean meat, poultry, fish, tofu
- Dried peas and beans, lentils, other legumes
- Nuts, seeds

Limit Saturated Fats for Memory

Your child needs an adequate intake of healthy fats, but too much fat, especially saturated fats, may impair their cognitive flexibility (the ability to think on their feet). This seems to be especially true when task demands increase, according to a study published in the scientific journal *Appetite*.[1] Saturated fats include butter, lard, hydrogenated oils and other fats that remain solid at room temperature. Choose these types of fats sparingly.

It's Your Pick!

If your child continually brings home a lunch pail that's barely touched, it's time to join forces. Picky eaters tend to eat more when they do the picking.

If your child is a picky eater, enlist their help. Invite your child to pick one food in the four main food groups—a vegetable, a fruit, a protein-rich food and a food rich in complex carbohydrates.

Don't forget to include a "drink pick" as well as a special treat or a "fun pick." Your child will feel valued that you are listening, and you'll be pleased to know that nourishing foods are fueling the day's learning. Read on to learn more about each "pick" list.

Parent Pearl

Use your imagination. My daughter has come up with all sorts of combinations for her lunch pail from apple slices with cinnamon to her own stackable creations with whole wheat crackers, cheese and luncheon meat. I have learned that my fussy eater will eat much more when she feels in charge of lunch.

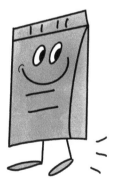

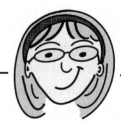

Did You Know?

If the newest sugar-laden cereal, high-fat snack or calorie-packed treat is just too enticing for your kids, establish a "dessert only" rule. Serve it up as an occasional dessert treat. The kids won't feel deprived, and you'll be helping keep their sugar intake to a minimum.

Vegetable Picks (phytonutrient-rich)

- Broccoli, cauliflower, jicama or other veggies cut into bite-size pieces
- Baby carrots (pre-washed and ready-to-go to save time during the early morning rush) or shredded carrot in a tuna sandwich
- Cherry tomatoes (rich in heart-healthy lycopene, and a beautiful and tasty combination when mixed with blueberries)
- Cucumbers
- Seaweed (can be found in convenient single-serving portions)
- Soybeans (often found in the frozen section; toss into a plastic bag in the morning to perfectly defrost for snack or lunchtime)
- Snap beans (kids love these little treasures)
- Sweet bell pepper (cut in strips)
- And many, many more!

Parent Pearl

Check out your local kitchen tool supply shop. There are all sorts of utensils available to turn the shape of plain old carrot and celery sticks into fancy stars or other fun shapes.

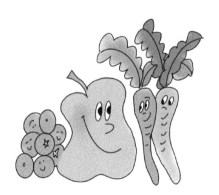

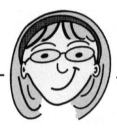

Did You Know?

Kids prefer vegetables cut into smaller pieces because they look less intimidating. You can tap into this natural preference to entice your child to eat more, even at school lunch. Pack colorful, bite-sized vegetables with a small container of hummus or other healthy dip, and your child is sure to start munching more.

Fruit Picks (phytonutrient-rich)

- Apple
- Applesauce (no sugar added)
- Banana
- Blueberries and other berries
- Cherries
- Fruit cocktail (packed in natural juices)
- Grapes
- Mandarin orange
- Melon chunks (you name it—cantaloupe, honeydew, watermelon, cassava)
- Orange slices
- Peach slices
- Pear
- Pineapple slices
- Plums
- Raisins
- Strawberries
- Tangerine
- And many, many more!

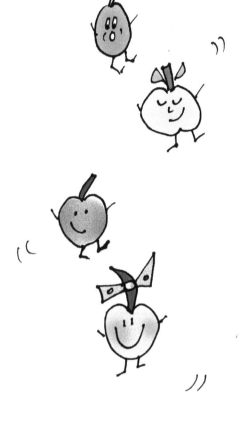

Note: It's best to avoid fruit roll ups since these choices stick to teeth and increase the risk of tooth decay and cavities.

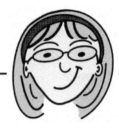

Did You Know?

You can help increase your child's fruit intake by choosing smaller pieces of fruit when shopping. Too often a big, delicious apple gets one bite and then is thrown away because the playground calls.

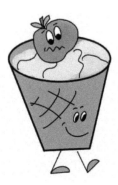

Protein Picks (aids alertness)

- Beans
- Beef jerky
- Cheese
- Chili
- Cottage cheese
- Falafel
- Grilled chicken/chicken strips
- Hard-boiled egg
- Nuts, seeds
- Peanut butter (the natural-type) or other nut butters such as cashew, almond or soy (combine with 100% fruit spread, sliced apple or banana, or raisins)
- Stew
- Trail mix (buy a big bag and place small portions into snack-size plastic bags)
- Tuna or salmon (rich in omega-3 fats)
- Turkey, chicken, ham or other low-fat or non-fat luncheon meat
- Yogurt (plain or flavored)

Parent Pearl

Bento boxes have a clever design that keeps foods separate in packed lunches. I pack a sandwich, pasta or salad in the bottom section, and nuts, seeds, crackers and more in the top section. There's even a separate space for dressing or dips. My kids (and their friends) always enjoy seeing what's inside! ☺

Carbohydrate Picks (for sustained energy)

- Bagel
- Cereal (consider a handful of cereal in a bag)
- Crackers
- English muffin
- Granola bar (choose whole grain bars portioned for kids)
- Muffins (make your own with your child's favorite additions like sunflower seeds, walnuts, raisins, cranberries, flax, shredded carrots or applesauce and store in the freezer. (Pack one during morning lunch prep, and it will be perfectly thawed by lunch)
- Pasta such as macaroni, noodles, spaghetti and others
- Pita chips
- Pita pockets (fill to the brim with sprouts, cucumbers, tomatoes and other fresh vegetables. Include a slice of cheese and/or luncheon meat for a protein boost)
- Pizza
- Popcorn
- Pretzel (and peanut butter dip)
- Rice and rice cakes
- Sandwich
- Soup (fill a thermos full of your child's favorite veggie or bean soup—a hit on a cold, blustery day)
- Starchy vegetables such as potato, corn, beans and peas
- Whole grain bread and rolls (pair up with hummus or cheese)
- Whole wheat tortillas (make a wrap with beans, cheese, turkey or chicken and top with tomato, avocado, pepper or cheese, or make a quesadilla with cheese)

Parent Pearl

Make enough for leftovers. When preparing dinners, I make extra pasta or other main dishes. The leftovers are a great (and easy) addition to my child's packed lunch for the next day.

Drink Picks (hydration boosters)

- Fruit juice such as apple, aronia, blueberry, boysenberry and pomegranate (consider adding a little sparkling water—approximately 3 parts juice to one part water—to make your own better-for-you soda)
- Fruit smoothie in a thermos
- Lemonade
- Milk (white or flavored)
- Rice milk
- Soy milk
- Vegetable juice
- Water

Note: Avoid fruit drinks, which are nothing more than refined sugar. Consider limiting fruit juice to no more than ½ to ¾ cup per day for young children, age 1 to 6 years old, and no more than 1 to 1½ cups daily for older kids. Although fruit juices contain natural unrefined sugar, they're lacking hunger-curbing fiber. A better choice is whole fruit.

Parent Pearl

Consider buying a thermos or two. Over the course of the school year, this one purchase has saved me a bundle. With two, I always have one ready to use if the other is in the dishwasher. It also saves time during our hectic school mornings.

Fun Picks (for a special treat)

Lunch is always so much sweeter when you open your lunch box to find a fun surprise. Consider writing a love note, joke, riddle, drawing or brainteaser on your child's napkin. Sports clips and comics are also great to include to encourage reading. What's more, your child's friends are likely to look forward to finding out what's inside the "fun" lunch pail.

Plan ahead and collect a stash of fun riddles and jokes from books or online sources. You'll avoid feeling stressed for time, and it will be a cinch to regularly include one in your child's lunch pail for a fun little extra to enjoy at lunch time.

Parent Pearl

Make fun sandwich shapes with cookie cutters. I reach for my heart-shaped cookie cutter to shape my kids' sandwiches into a special surprise just to say, "I love you!"

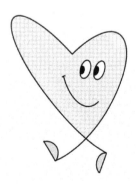

This Month's Smart Goal

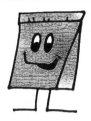

I will have my child help with the planning and making of school lunches at least once a week.

This Month's Extra Credit

I will include a joke, riddle, brainteaser or other fun pick in my child's lunch box at least twice a week.

To monitor your daily progress toward your goals, use the **My Smart Tracker** forms in **Chapter 14: Go for the Goal.**

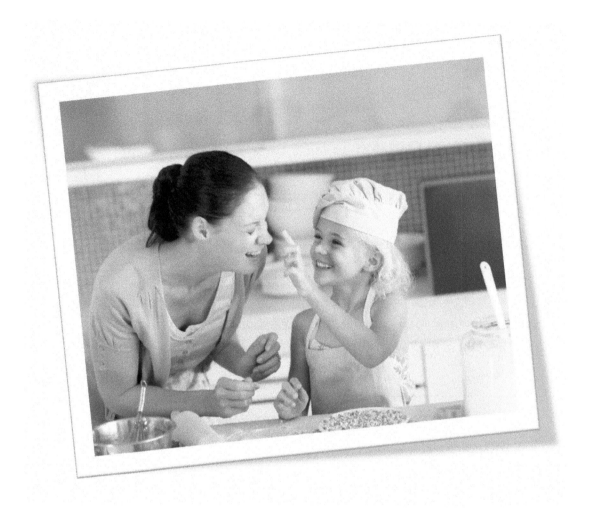

Find something you're passionate about
and keep tremendously interested in it.
— Julia Child

Chapter 7

February – Kids in the Kitchen

Exposing your child to an enriching environment is one of the best ways to sharpen their mind. What fits the bill better than cooking in the kitchen? Cracking an egg can challenge dexterity while providing an opportune time to talk to your child about choline, the brain-building nutrient found in eggs. You can challenge math skills by asking your child to double the ingredients in a favorite cookie recipe. Let your child convert kitchen equivalents—3 teaspoons per tablespoon, 2 cups per pint and 16 ounces per pound. You can even ask your child to read a recipe aloud to build confidence in public speaking. Even the very littlest helper can join in on the kitchen fun. Give them pots, pans and spoons to pretend to measure out an ingredient or even bang out a happy kitchen tune. The opportunities are endless, and your time is well spent. After all, taking the time to teach children to cook not only helps build a skill for life, but it also gives them an opportunity to share what's really going on in their lives.

The checklists that follow will help you choose age-appropriate tasks that are sure to inspire your child's inner chef—one step at a time.

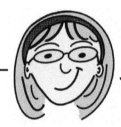

Did You Know?

Cooking with your child is the perfect time to practice volumes. Use measuring cups and spoons that are clearly marked to help reinforce equivalent measures. Here are a few common equivalents to get you started:

3 teaspoons = 1 tablespoon
16 tablespoons = 1 cup
2 cups = 1 pint
2 pints = 1 quart
4 quarts = 1 gallon

Inspiring Your Child's Inner Chef
(Kindergarten to 3rd Grade)

Check (☑) the box for each task your child has already tried. Place an X (☒) in the box for each new task to try.

❑ Adding ingredients

❑ Dropping cookie dough on trays

❑ Frosting cupcakes

❑ Husking corn (tiny fingers are perfectly suited to remove the hairs from the cob)

❑ Kneading dough

❑ Peeling hard boiled eggs

❑ Pouring cold liquids

❑ Reading recipes out loud

❑ Rolling dough

❑ Shelling peas

❑ Spreading peanut butter or jelly on bread

❑ Stirring

❑ Tearing lettuce into pieces for a salad

❑ Washing fruits and veggies

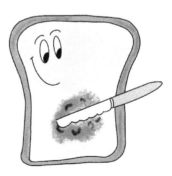

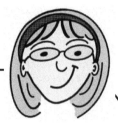

Did You Know?

You can help keep everyone safe in the kitchen while you enjoy cooking by following a few simple rules:

1. Use aprons.
2. Avoid wearing baggy clothes, including shirts with long, loose sleeves.
3. Put long hair back in a ponytail.
4. For older children, establish an age-appropriate "no touch" rule for knives and other sharp utensils; for younger children, keep sharp utensils away and out of sight.
5. At the stove, keep the handles of pots and pans away from the edge, turning them inward toward the stove.
6. Cook hot foods on the back burners, if possible.
7. Always supervise when fire or knives are in use.
8. Turn off the stove when finished.

Inspiring Your Child's Inner Chef
(4th Grade to 6th Grade)

> *Check (☑) the box for each task your child has already tried. Place an X (☒) in the box for each new task to try.*

- ❑ Cracking eggs; separating whites from yolks
- ❑ Cutting fruits and veggies
- ❑ Filling muffin tins
- ❑ Helping to plan meals
- ❑ Helping to modify a recipe
- ❑ Measuring and mixing ingredients
- ❑ Peeling vegetables
- ❑ Reading food labels
- ❑ Reading recipes out loud
- ❑ Setting the table
- ❑ Using the can opener, blender and microwave
- ❑ Using a whisk
- ❑ Washing dishes

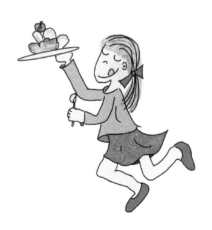

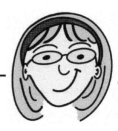

Did You Know?

Smell is one of our most powerful senses and can trigger memories from decades ago. Think of how the sweet smell of fresh citrus can bring you back to a childhood romp through an orange grove, or how the smell of freshly cut grass reminds you of a sunny afternoon playing in a park.

You can help your child form these same feel-good memories by using aromatic foods in your recipes—cookies made with pure vanilla, bread baked with fresh rosemary or lemonade juiced from whole lemons.

10 Tips for Cooking Success

Make your time in the kitchen a smashing success with these easy-to-use tips:

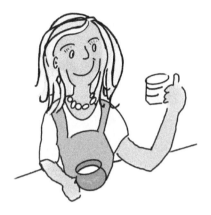

1 **Loosen up.** The key to any successful cooking adventure is to choose a time when you're both relaxed. An ideal time would be a lazy weekend morning or a weekday afternoon after homework is finished. Block off your calendar, turn up the music and have fun.

2 **Ask your child to read the recipe to you.** This will help ensure that each step is understood before beginning and that no emergency runs to the grocery store are needed.

3 **Safety at all times.** Set ground rules to emphasize the importance of safety. Teach kindergartners to avoid touching hot stovetops and pans, whirring blenders and sharp knife blades. Discuss what's OK to touch and what's off limits. Remind older children as well. Safety will go a long way toward making the most of your special kitchen time.

4 **Scrub-a-dub-dub.** Before working with food, make sure all little hands are properly washed. Here's how: Wet hands under warm water, lather up with soap, wash for at least 30 seconds and rinse. To keep track of time, sing the alphabet song (it's just about the right amount of time to ensure a thorough cleaning). If a recipe calls for meat, fish or poultry, be sure to also wash hands immediately after handling.

5 **Clean as you go.** An uncluttered kitchen makes for a more enjoyable experience. Teach your youngster to put containers of food back as you use them and to clean up as you go. This not only keeps your space free of clutter as you cook, but will also make cleaning up at the end a breeze.

6 **Fresh is best.** Use the freshest ingredients possible. We can't stress this enough. The wonderful aromas and flavors lend an irresistible joy to handling ingredients that are at their seasonal peak like a tomato plucked from the vine, a fresh sprig of dill or a pineapple bursting with juice.

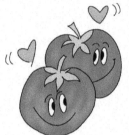

7 **Cut the fat and sugar; boost the fiber.** Most likely, your treasured recipes rely on fat or sugar for a flavorful impact. Yet, it may only take a slight adjustment to make them healthier without affecting the flavors that your family loves. For recipe makeover ideas, check out **Recipe Makeover Tips & Tricks** on page 275.

8 **Be prepared.** Don't leave your cupboards bare. Be ready for whipping up a quick meal before your child's hunger strikes or if unexpected guests drop by. For inspiration to get started, check out **Stocking Your Fridge, Freezer & Pantry** on page 279.

9 **Tools of the trade.** Having the proper kitchen tools on hand can make the difference between enjoying your time in the kitchen and dreading it. For a list of need-to-haves (and a few nice-to-haves), check out **Choosing Kitchen Utensils & Tools** on page 282.

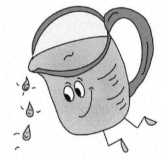

10 **Praise.** There will be spills and messes as you go. It's just part of the learning process. Take it in stride and enjoy your precious time together. When you catch your child doing something right, be ready with praise (the more specific, the better). In this way, you'll help build your child's self-esteem and increase the odds that they'll want to spend more time in the kitchen. Who knows, you might have a future master chef in the making!

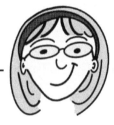

Did You Know?

American's Test Kitchen Kids provides a variety of activities for your budding chef. Here you'll find an assortment of free kid-friendly recipes, hands-on activities, books, subscription boxes, a YouTube® channel and more. You'll even find a Mystery Recipe podcast for a fun way to learn about cooking. Learn more at www.americastestkitchen.com/kids.

Vocabulary-Building Cooking

Build vocabulary while you cook. Here's how: Grab an ingredient, and ask your child to describe it using one-word adjectives. Choose words using all the senses—sight, smell, touch, taste and hearing. Check out the list below for inspiration.

acidic   appealing   appetizing   aromatic   astringent   bitter

bland   brittle   bumpy   buttery   burnt   chewy   chilly

citrus   cold   crisp   crystals   crunchy   crusty   delicious

delectable   delightful   doughy   dry   earthy   flavorsome

flat   fluid   frosty   frozen   glossy   gooey   gummy   hard

healthy   heavy   hot   icy   juicy   leathery   light   luscious

lukewarm   liquid   long   melting   mild   moist   mouth-

watering   mushy   musty   peppery   plump   pungent

rough   round   salty   savory   scrumptious   sharp   shiny

slick   slushy   smoky   smooth   soggy   soft   sour   spicy

spotted   sticky   stringy   strong   succulent   sugary   sweet

syrupy   tangy   tart   tasteless   tasty   tender   tough

tepid   vinegary   viscous   warm   wet   weak   wilted

yeasty   yucky   yummy   zesty

Fill Your Plate for Performance

Teach your child how to fill their plate with foods that give them energy and enhance performance. Here's how:

1 Ask your child to look at their plate and draw an imaginary line down the middle.

2 Explain that one half of the plate is devoted to non-starchy veggies such as spinach, tomatoes, carrots, zucchini and beets, just to name a few.

3 Once filled, ask your child to draw another imaginary line down the center of the empty half of the plate. Explain that one part is for protein-rich foods such as fish, chicken, meat or tofu, and the other part is for grains or starchy foods.

4 Top the meal off with a glass of milk and a piece of fruit, and your child is ready to conquer their world.

You can even add some fun to the learning process with the **Rate Your Plate Game** on page 127.

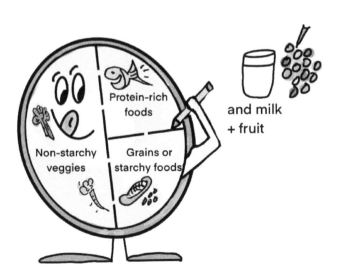

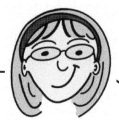

Did You Know?

You can teach your child to set the table like a pro in six easy steps. Here's how:

1. Place the plate in the center.
2. To the left, add the forks. If a salad fork is needed, place it to the far left since it's used first.
3. To the right, place the knife (blade toward the plate) and the spoon to the far right.
4. Slide the plate to one inch from the edge of table.
5. Add a napkin under the fork(s) or on the plate.
6. Finish by adding a cup to the upper right of the setting.

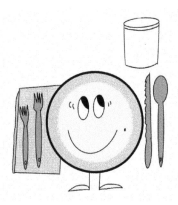

Rate Your Plate Game

Rate Your Plate is a fun game to help your child learn about healthy food choices and proper serving sizes. Get the entire family involved. The rules are simple. Check out the five healthy choices below. Each one earns one or more points. Whoever scores the most points is the mealtime winner!

1 point for <u>each</u> fruit or vegetable

1 point for <u>each</u> fruit or vegetable of a
    different color

1 point for a milk, cheese or other dairy product

1 point for a whole grain food

1 point for a protein-rich food

Parent Pearl

I love my pannini press. It's so easy to make an extra tasty sandwich, while at the same time packing in plenty of veggies. The flavors blend so well, and the kids often ask for more!

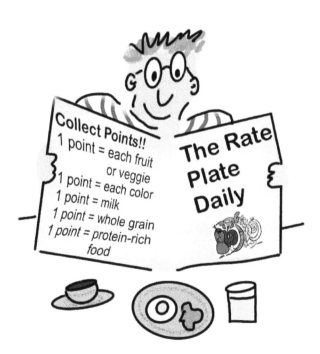

Collect Points!!
1 point = each fruit or veggie
1 point = each color
1 point = milk
1 point = whole grain
1 point = protein-rich food

The Rate Plate Daily

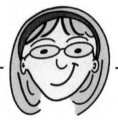

Did You Know?

The nutrition experts at the Academy of Nutrition and Dietetics provide handy resources for reliable information about the unique nutrient needs and physical activity recommendations for grade-school children 6 to 12 years of age. Here you'll find articles about healthy meals and snacks, food allergies and intolerances, ideas to be active and more, all designed to help you nourish your child's inner awesomeness. To learn more, visit www.eatright.org.

The Apple Doesn't Fall Far from the Tree

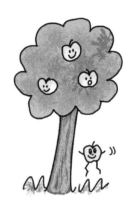

If you have a picky eater, look at yourself. Picky eating may be a genetic trait. Studies report certain people have a genetic sensitivity to a bitter food compound called 6-n-propylthiouracil or PROP for short. The ability to taste PROP may play a role in a child's love-it or hate-it approach to broccoli, spinach, cabbage, Brussels sprouts and other bitter-tasting vegetables. What's more, kids who are PROP tasters are also reported to be more sensitive to sweet and pungent tastes as well as to the texture of fats.[1]

Is your child a super taster?

If your child is a picky eater, they may be a super taster and bitter flavors may be their kryptonite. Well, wonder no more, thanks to PTC tasting strips, a favorite of science teachers for lessons that demonstrate the effects of heredity on taste.

PTC stands for phenylthiourea, a compound that mimics the bitterness of broccoli, Brussels sprouts and other cruciferous veggies. Have your child place a strip on their tongue, you'll know right away whether they're genetically predisposed to being a super taster (it will be intensely bitter). You'll also know that you're not crazy, your child really does taste differently than other people.

Parent Pearl

Let the kids cook.
Once a month, I let the kids choose a meal to make. Their creations are incredible, plus it's priceless to see the smile on their face from a job well done.

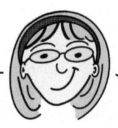

Did You Know?

Kids (like all of us) learn best by doing. When teaching your child a new skill in the kitchen, the wisdom of three applies:

1. First, let your child observe what you are doing.
2. Next, let your child do the same activity with your coaching, offering encouragement and guidance.
3. Finally, let your child try it solo.

Tips to Entice PROP Tasters

If your child is a PROP taster, they're sure to be super sensitive to bitter flavors and likely have some sensitivity to overly sweet and pungent flavors. However, don't get discouraged. To help entice their discriminating palette, consider one or more of these food preparation tips:

- Stir-fry or otherwise lightly cook broccoli, cabbage and other bitter veggies to reduce the bitter bite.
- Grate, mince or puree carrots, zucchini, spinach and other veggies into pasta sauces, soups and quiches. The more you blend them, the less your child will recognize them.
- Lightly sweeten winter squash, carrots and other root vegetables with honey or brown sugar.
- Neutralize the taste of bitter salad greens with avocado or a little olive oil. Some bitter compounds dissolve when mixed with fats.
- Offer a dip or dressing with veggies.
- Sprinkle raw veggies with lemon juice or balsamic vinegar.
- Add a pinch of salt to veggies to help block the bitterness and enhance the sweetness.

Parent Pearl

To speed up meal prep when measuring spoons are missing, I simply use my thumb as a guide. From tip to first knuckle, your thumb is about one teaspoon. Simply multiply by three and you have a tablespoon.

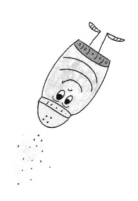

This Month's Smart Goal

I will have my child help create one complete meal for the family this month (grocery shopping, cooking and setting the table).

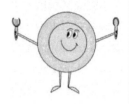

This Month's Extra Credit

I will play Rate Your Plate with my child at three meals per week (and earn at least 5 points per session).

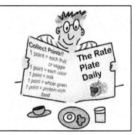

To monitor your daily progress toward your goals, use the **My Smart Tracker** forms in **Chapter 14: Go for the Goal.**

Part 4

Spring Fever

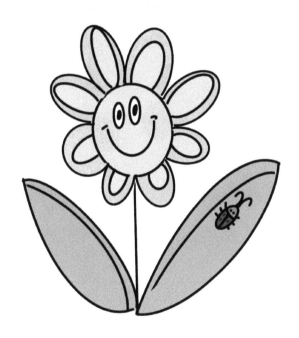

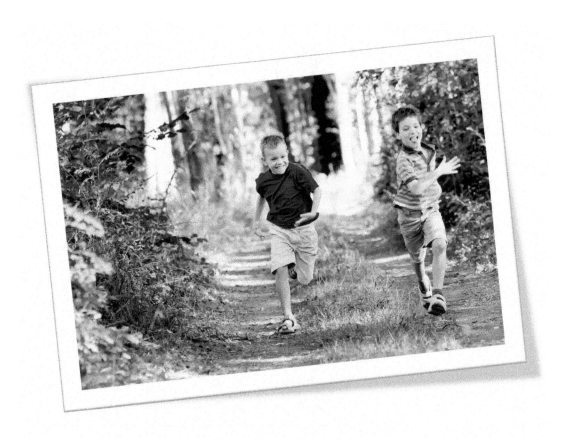

Genius is 1 percent inspiration
and 99 percent perspiration.
— Thomas Edison

Chapter 8

March – Fit Body, Fit Brain

If you think your child can fully exercise their brain just by studying, think again. Physical activity is also essential. By increasing blood flow to the brain, physical activity helps deliver life-sustaining oxygen as well as glucose, the brain's preferred energy source.

Physical activity also triggers the production of chemicals, called nerve growth factors, which appear to extend the life of brain cells and increase their number and the connections between them. Activity also activates brain cells to release serotonin and norepinephrine, two important biochemical messengers that help sustain attention and the ability to concentrate. The result: A brain that's more efficient and adaptive, which translates into better learning and performance for your child.

By 6 years of age, blood flow and oxygen consumption in a child's brain achieve staggeringly high rates, the highest of any life stage. At this age, the brain's oxygen consumption corresponds to more than 50% of the body's total intake, a rate that gradually declines until adulthood.[1] Researchers have yet to pinpoint why this extraordinarily high metabolic rate occurs in a child's brain, but they do know one thing. All that growth and development requires plenty of oxygen, a steady supply of glucose and an optimal flow of blood to deliver what a child's active brain needs.

What Exercise Is Best?

Physical activity is the best way to get the heart pumping and blood flowing throughout the body and brain. Just about any activity will help increase blood flow to the brain. What's more, there's no shortage of enjoyable activities available to your child such as swinging on the monkey bars, jumping rope or playing hopscotch, just to name a few.

The trick is to encourage your child to choose something they enjoy. It could be an individual activity, team sport or simply free play. For ideas to include more fun activities in your child's life, check out **Fitness from A to Z** list on page 138.

Parent Pearl

Step it up. My son loves his pedometer. He keeps track of his daily steps and is delighted when he breaks a new record. Being the competitive type, he also loves to challenge the rest of the family to a "step off," which helps keep everyone more active.

How Much Exercise?

There are 1,440 minutes in a day. The U.S. Department of Health & Human Services recommends school-aged children spend at least 60 of them engaged in some type of moderate to vigorous activity.[2] This level of physical activity not only supports your child's brain health and academic performance, but it also promotes a higher fitness level, lower body fat, stronger bones and muscles and even a more positive outlook and brighter mood.

For some kids, this can feel like an easy target. For others, it can seem like a daunting goal. If your child sweats at the mere thought of exercise, be sure to take it slowly with small goals. And, above all, make it extra fun. After all, kids love to play, so approach exercise as play.

As your child gets into better shape, their ability to move with greater coordination and agility is sure to bring a welcome surge in self-esteem and confidence, along with lots of smiles. Remember, you're helping to build a healthy habit that your child will take into adulthood (and likely pass on to their kids).

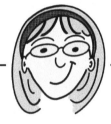

Did You Know?

Active video games (also known as exergames) are so much more than just good fun. These games are a promising tool to help kids stay physically fit, according to one meta-analysis published in the July 2021 issue of the *International Journal of Environmental Research and Public Health*. The researchers found these digital games not only help kids maintain a healthy body mass index (BMI) and improve heart health and lung function, but also appear to be a great way to help kids fine-tune their motor skills.[3]

Fitness from A to Z

> Check (☑) the box next to the activity that sounds like fun to your child.
> Choose one to try today.

- ❑ Aerobics
- ❑ Badminton
- ❑ Baseball
- ❑ Basketball
- ❑ Bowling
- ❑ Climbing
- ❑ Cycling
- ❑ Dance
- ❑ Dodge-Ball
- ❑ Duck, Duck, Goose
- ❑ Equestrian Events
- ❑ Football
- ❑ Four Square
- ❑ Free Play
- ❑ Frisbee
- ❑ Golf
- ❑ Gymnastics
- ❑ Handball
- ❑ Hiking
- ❑ Hockey
- ❑ Hopscotch
- ❑ Hula Hooping

- ❑ Ice Skating
- ❑ Inline Skating
- ❑ Jump Roping
- ❑ Kickball
- ❑ Kite Flying
- ❑ Lacrosse
- ❑ Martial Arts
- ❑ Monkey Bars
- ❑ Nature Walk
- ❑ Off-Road Biking
- ❑ Outdoor Activities
- ❑ Playing Catch
- ❑ Quidditch
- ❑ Red Light, Green Light
- ❑ Roller-skating
- ❑ Running
- ❑ Shuffleboard
- ❑ Skateboarding
- ❑ Skiing
- ❑ Snorkeling
- ❑ Snowboarding
- ❑ Soccer

- ❑ Softball
- ❑ Swimming
- ❑ Table Tennis
- ❑ Tag
- ❑ T-Ball
- ❑ Tennis
- ❑ Tetherball
- ❑ Ultimate Frisbee
- ❑ Volleyball
- ❑ Walking
- ❑ Xare (a racquetball game)
- ❑ YMCA activities
- ❑ Zoo Visit
- ❑ Zorbing (for the adventurous)

Others:
- ❑ _____
- ❑ _____
- ❑ _____
- ❑ _____

Five Ways to Encourage Regular Activity

1 **Walk to school.** Henry David Thoreau said it best, "An early-morning walk is a blessing for a whole day." If practical, walk your child to school. It has rewards well beyond physical activity: the giggles from seeing their face reflected in a puddle, the joy of discovering a new bug along the pathway or the delight of spotting a glorious sunflower smiling down from its high perch. Plus, you'll be making fond memories that will last a lifetime.

2 **Take charge.** Don't leave physical activity to the whims of others. Some schools or teachers may encourage enriching physical activities, but sadly, this is no longer the norm. Take charge by planning some of your family time around recreational activities like a hike, a bike ride or a friendly basketball game.

3 **Listen to your child.** Help your child choose an activity based on their temperament. Kids who thrive on competition and love interacting with others may prefer baseball, basketball, soccer, volleyball or another team sport. For kids who prefer a more individual challenge, activities such as cross-country running, singles tennis, martial arts or gymnastics may be a better choice. And, kids who go weak at the knees with the whole win/lose scenario may enjoy hiking, dancing, outdoor play or another activity that encourages a cooperative spirit.

4 **Don't overdo it.** Use the sing/talk test. If your child can sing while exercising, the activity may be too easy. If they can only say a few words without pausing to catch their breath, it may be too hard. The key is to find the right balance.

5 **Be a role model for good health.** If you want an active child, be active yourself. No amount of talking can ever replace the impact of watching a parent practice what they preach. Your example is the most powerful tool in your toolbox.

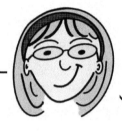

Did You Know?

Regular physical activity is directly linked to a child's academic performance, according to one meta-analysis[1] of 31 studies involving children between 6 and 12 years of age.

For this analysis, the researchers focused on the impact of physical activity on specific types of mental functions like memory, planning and other so-called executive functions, attention and academic performance in math, spelling and reading. Results are published in the May 2018 issue of the *Journal of Science and Medicine in Sport*.

The researchers found as little as one bout of activity had an immediate benefit on a child's ability to pay attention (think focusing in the classroom after playing at recess). Even better, when physical activity was on a regular basis, it improved all types of mental function: attention, executive function and academic performance. In other words, active kids who engage in regular activity are better able to focus, learn and excel in school.[4]

Fueling Active Kids for Competition

Now that your child is active, you may be wondering what to feed them before a soccer game, a long run or another intense activity. The good news is the types of foods that fuel your child's athletic performance are the same as those that fuel their brain for peak mental performance. The only difference is in the timing.

In general, kids need to eat small meals throughout the day to optimize energy. When it comes to physical activity—especially intense training sessions, competitive games and other extremely vigorous activities—consider feeding your child according to the time intervals outlined below.[5,6]

Three or four hours before a game or practice

Three to four hours before an activity, have your child fill up on a carbohydrate-rich meal. For breakfast, consider oatmeal with slices of banana and a sprinkle of cinnamon, whole grain toast and a cup of steamy hot chocolate. For lunch, consider a turkey and veggie sandwich, milk and a piece of fruit. For dinner, consider a dish of marinara pasta with a sprinkle of cheese, a green salad, crisp apple slices and milk.

One hour before a game or practice

One hour before an activity, offer your child a snack. Consider a granola bar, four or five graham crackers, a half a bagel or a banana. It's also important for your child to be well hydrated. Make sure they drink at least 1½ cups (12 ounces) of water at this time.

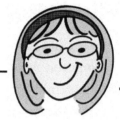

Did You Know?

If your child has more than one competitive athletic match during the same day, it's especially important to refuel between matches. A good rule of thumb is to eat 0.7 grams of carbohydrates per pound of body weight no later than 30 minutes after a match. For example, if your child weighs 75 pounds, a snack or meal with at least 53 grams of carbs is ideal. Here are a few kid-friendly options to consider:

Food	Carbohydrates
Apple (1 small)	15 grams
Orange (1 small)	15 grams
Banana (1 small)	15 grams
Berries (1 cup)	15 grams
Juice (½ cup)	15 grams
Sweet or white potato (3 ounces)	15 grams
Bread (1 slice)	15 grams
Bagel (¼ each or 1 ounce)	15 grams
Milk (1 cup)	12 grams
Yogurt (¾ cup)	12 grams
Granola or energy bar (1 each)	Varies (check label)
Sports drink (1 each)	Varies (check label)

During a game or practice

Keep the water flowing! Water is the best choice during and after a workout to rehydrate. Sports drinks are another popular option. They typically contain sodium and other electrolytes that can be lost in sweat during prolonged, vigorous activity. But, the sugar-acid combo typical of sports drinks can dramatically increase the risk of tooth decay and other dental issues. Be sure to keep water handy for a quick rinse. And, for less intense activity, water is best.

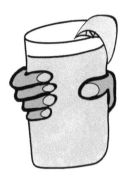

After a game or practice

After activity, it's time to rehydrate and refuel. Have your child drink plenty of water. A good rule of thumb is to drink about 2 cups (16 ounces) of water for every pound of body weight lost. In addition, have your child eat a carbohydrate-rich food within 30 minutes after the end of the workout. This is especially important for a competitive player who has more rounds of competition later the same day. It helps replenish the body's glycogen stores to fuel the next performance. Here, timing is key, so don't wait too long. The muscles are especially primed to store glycogen within 30 minutes after a vigorous bout of activity.

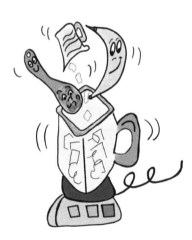

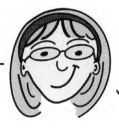

Did You Know?

Kids who spend more time outside during daylight hours are less likely to be nearsighted. The eye grows throughout childhood, but if it grows too long from front to back, the result is nearsightedness (myopia) and blurry distance vision that could require glasses.

Researchers believe the unique features of sunlight help prevent myopia, especially its intensity. With an intensity hundreds of times higher than that of indoor lighting, sunlight stimulates the release of dopamine in the retina. This, in turn, works to prevent a child's eyeball from growing too long. Plus, sunlight shrinks the pupils, deepens the depth of field, and reduces blurring, all factors that may help prevent myopia.

Whatever the reason, one thing is clear: Spending time outdoors in full daylight is not only good for your child's body and brain, it's good for their eyesight. For this reason, optometrists recommend children 6 years of age and older spend at least 2 hours every day outside in the sunshine.[7]

The Cost of Physical Inactivity

Regular physical activity plays a key role in helping your child maintain a healthy body weight, excel in school and build self-confidence. Conversely, physical inactivity and excess body weight have profound negative effects that sap the body, mind and spirit.

An analysis of data from a national survey of children's health[8] involving more than 22,900 children tells the story. For this study, researchers were interested in the link between body mass index (BMI) and five key markers of academic skills and coping strategies. The markers included whether a child does all their required homework, shows interest and curiosity in learning new things, works to finish tasks they start, stays calm and in control when faced with a challenge, and cares about doing well in school. In other words, how well a child is flourishing.

After correcting for potential confounding variables like age, depression, sleep, digital media exposure and others, the researchers found only 29% of the kids with a BMI in the obese range had all five flourishing markers compared to about 40% of kids with a BMI in the normal or overweight range. Results are published in the January 2021 issue of the *Journal of Pediatrics*. While more research is needed to confirm these findings, this study offers keen insight into the potential link between a child's BMI and their ability to thrive in school and face challenging situations.

What's a parent to do? First and foremost, be a role model and keep the lines of communication open. Next, continue to reinforce healthy habits with tools such as this book. Finally, reach out for additional resources. With childhood obesity at an all-time high (more than 35% of kids and teens in the United States are now overweight or obese[9]), experts are increasing their efforts to address this serious public health concern. As a result, more resources and tools are likely to be available to help families, schools and communities tackle childhood obesity.

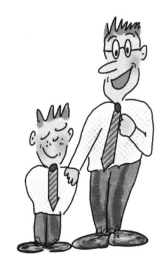

Is Your Child's Weight Healthy?

Body mass index (BMI) is generally a good predicator of overall health. It uses your child's weight and height to estimate body fat. To calculate your child's BMI, use an online tool like the BMI Percentile Calculator for Child and Teen by the Centers for Disease Control and Prevention (www.cdc.gov), or calculate it using the steps below.

Step 1: Weigh your child and enter the amount in pounds below:

_____ (my child's weight in pounds)

Step 2: Measure your child's height in inches and enter the amount below:

_____ (my child's height in inches)

Step 3: Calculate your child's BMI using the following formula:

BMI = [weight ÷ (height)^2] x 703.

For example, a 50-pound child who is 48 inches tall has a BMI of 15.3:

BMI = [weight ÷ (height)^2] x 703

BMI = [50 pounds ÷ (48 inches)^2] x 703

BMI = [50 pounds ÷ 2,304] x 703

BMI = 15.3

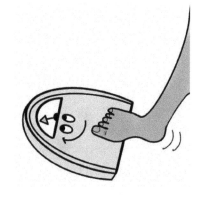

My child's BMI is:

BMI = [_____ pounds ÷ (_____ inches)^2] x 703

BMI = _____

Step 4: Select the BMI chart below for your child (girl or boy). Find your child's age and determine which weight category the BMI falls into (i.e., underweight, healthy weight, overweight or obese).

Body Mass Index (BMI) Categories for Children				
Age	**Underweight**	**Healthy BMI**	**Overweight**	**Obese**
For Boys				
5 years	less than 13.9	13.9 up to 16.8	16.8 up to 17.8	17.8 or more
6 years	less than 13.8	13.8 up to 16.9	16.9 up to 18.1	18.1 or more
7 years	less than 13.7	13.7 up to 17.2	17.2 up to 18.8	18.8 or more
8 years	less than 13.7	13.7 up to 17.7	17.7 up to 19.6	19.6 or more
9 years	less than 13.9	13.9 up to 18.3	18.3 up to 20.6	20.6 or more
10 years	less than 14.1	14.1 up to 19.0	19.0 up to 21.6	21.6 or more
11 years	less than 14.4	14.4 up to 19.8	19.8 up to 22.7	22.7 or more
12 years	less than 14.8	14.8 up to 20.6	20.6 up to 23.7	23.7 or more
For Girls				
5 years	less than 13.5	13.5 up to 16.8	16.8 up to 18.2	18.2 or more
6 years	less than 13.4	13.4 up to 17.1	17.1 up to 18.8	18.8 or more
7 years	less than 13.4	13.4 up to 17.6	17.6 up to 19.6	19.6 or more
8 years	less than 13.5	13.5 up to 18.3	18.3 up to 20.6	20.6 or more
9 years	less than 13.7	13.7 up to 19.0	19.0 up to 21.7	21.7 or more
10 years	less than 14.0	14.0 up to 19.9	19.9 up to 22.9	22.9 or more
11 years	less than 14.4	14.4 up to 20.8	20.8 up to 24.0	24.0 or more
12 years	less than 14.8	14.8 up to 21.7	21.7 up to 25.2	25.2 or more
Source: Centers for Disease Control and Prevention (www.cdc.gov)				

How Many Calories Are Enough?

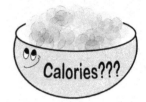

The number of calories your child needs to maintain a healthy body weight depends on a variety of factors such as their activity level, age, height and weight. Counting calories is generally not necessary, but knowing a ballpark number may help you plan a healthy diet. Remember to include a wide variety of nutritious foods from each food group in order to optimize mental and physical performance. You'll find details about your child's calorie and food needs in **Chapter 15: Tables, Tips & More**. Focus on two tables: **Recommended Daily Intake: Calories** on page 286 and **Recommended Daily Intake: Food Groups** on page 289.

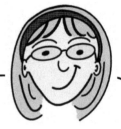

Did You Know?

It's important to serve your child age-appropriate portions because children take cues from their parents to decide how much to eat (like the amount of food you serve them). Serve larger portions, and your child is likely to eat too much and gain too much weight. Children also rely on their own internal hunger and satiety cues to self-regulate their food intake to match their needs (all healthy children are born with this innate ability). Allowing your child to choose their own portion size and rely on their internal cues to gauge their level of hunger or fullness is a self-reliance skill they can use to avoid eating too much now and in the future, when they are more independent and eat away from home more.[10]

Watch Out for Portion Distortion

Studies show our ability to judge the amount of food on our plate is affected by the size of the plate we use. A portion of food will appear smaller and more compact when it's served on a large, imposing plate. The same portion, however, will appear noticeably larger when served on a smaller plate. Why? Our brain makes a false assessment about the quantity of food. It's a visual illusion based on the principle of concentric circles.

In practical terms, the plate needs to be at least two-thirds full for your eye to feel satisfied. What does this mean for you and your child? If your child is overweight, consider using a smaller plate so they don't feel deprived. Conversely, if your child is a picky eater, consider using a larger plate so they don't feel overwhelmed with the amount of food on their plate.

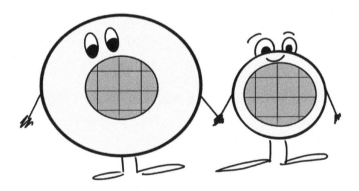

The principle of concentric circles. A portion of food will appear smaller and more compact when served on a large, imposing plate—a great choice to entice a picky eater. The same portion, however, will appear noticeably larger when served on a smaller plate— a great choice to help satisfy an overweight child.

Five Activity Tips to Train the Brain for Greatness

1 **Join the exergaming craze.** This blend of technology and fitness transforms sedentary screen-time into physically active screen-time. Think dance floors, step games and other interactive games that help kids sharpen their mental (and motor) skills, all while having fun. Dance games continue to be a favorite among young kids and are available for PlayStation, Xbox, Nintendo, and other popular brands of video game consoles.

2 **Watch the greats.** Watching someone else perform an action activates the brain in a similar way as performing the action yourself. It's called "action observation," and it's a common training technique to sharpen motor skills. Even better, combine it with the next tip for more mental muscle to fine-tune sports skills.[11]

3 **If you can imagine it, you can be it.** Tap into the technique of visualization to help stimulate the brain. For example, if your child wants to learn basketball, encourage using the "mind's eye" to see the ball going into the hoop, hear the swoosh as it rolls around, and experience the applause of the crowd. The more vivid the imagination, the stronger the effect.[12]

4 **Use your head, don't hurt your brain.** Make sure your child has proper protection when participating in various activities. For example, ensure that helmets fit securely while cycling or playing football.

5 **Share a laugh.** Laughing stimulates the brain, so don't underestimate the value of the lighter side of life. Laugh a lot, and laugh often.

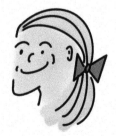

This Month's Smart Goal

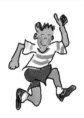

I will add 5 minutes of jumping, running or other fun activity until my child is active at least 60 minutes every day. (Take it one step at a time, listen to your child, and make sure it's fun.)

This Month's Extra Credit

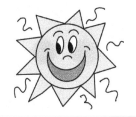

I will help my child play outside in full sunlight at least 2 hours each day to promote healthy vision.

To monitor your daily progress toward your goals, use the **My Smart Tracker** forms in **Chapter 14: Go for the Goal.**

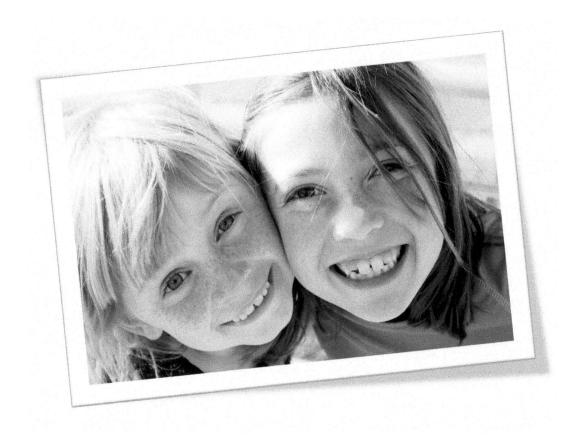

Nothing great was ever achieved without enthusiasm.
—Ralph Waldo Emerson

Chapter 9

April – Celebration beyond Cupcakes

With so many milestones to celebrate—birthdays, team victories, classroom achievements and more—your child is likely to be served plenty of cupcakes, cakes, cookies and similar sweets. In fact, no longer are these foods a small treat after enjoying more nutrient-dense foods, they now command center stage at most celebrations.

Trouble is, these foods are typically loaded with sugar, a triple whammy for your child: Empty calories, tooth decay and brain drain. The good news is, with a little know-how, you can easily learn how to limit sugary foods and choose healthier options more often without putting a damper on all the fun.

Limit Empty Calories

With childhood obesity at an all-time high, it's more important than ever to focus on limiting your child's intake of sugary foods with empty calories. Not banish, just limit. Even nutrition experts say every healthy diet can include a few empty calories.

Aim for no more than 15% of your child's daily calorie intake in the form of empty calories (the fewer, the better). We call this the 15% Rule. In practical terms, this means no more than a few hundred calories each day (less than one typical frosting-laden cupcake). Keeping these empty calories under control is a great way to help your child maintain a healthy body weight. You'll find all the need-to-know details in **Recommenced Daily Intake: Calories** on page 286 and **Recommend Daily "Empty" Calorie Limit** on page 287.

Smile Saving Strategy

When you use the 15% Rule to limit the intake of sugary foods, you'll not only help your child maintain a healthy body weight, but also help protect their teeth. Why? One of the main causes of tooth decay (in children and adults) is the total amount of time teeth are exposed to sugar.

In the mouth, bacteria quickly transform sugar into acids that attack tooth enamel and cause tooth decay. Eating sugary foods throughout the day allows for plenty of acid-producing activity that can increase the risk of cavities. By contrast, the 15% Rule helps deny mouth bacteria the sugar it needs to do its dirty work. The result is likely to be fewer cavities and better dental checkups.

A Better Sweet for Your Sweetie

Some kids just love sweets. The trick is to find a healthier substitute that they love just as much. On the next page, you'll find ideas to inspire you to limit the cake, candy and other sugary or high-fat foods and reach more often for nutrient-dense alternatives that pack a flavor punch.

Frosted cake

- ❏ Blueberry Mini Muffins*
- ❏ Brainy Banana Bread*
- ❏ Fresh fruit kabobs with fruit-flavored yogurt dip
- ❏ Fruity Yogurt Parfait*
- ❏ Going Coconuts for Pineapple Cake*
- ❏ Yummy Crumbly Crisp*

Chewy candy

- ❏ 100% xylitol- or sorbitol-sweetened gum
- ❏ Chocolate bar (choose mini ones for easier portion control)
- ❏ Crackers with old-fashioned peanut butter
- ❏ Dried fruit (apricots, raisins, mangoes, plums and others)
- ❏ Fresh fruit
- ❏ Fruit and nut bar
- ❏ Granola or trail mix
- ❏ Whole grain bar

Cookies

- ❏ Animal crackers
- ❏ Gingersnaps
- ❏ Graham crackers
- ❏ Unsweetened fruit-nut-seed bar
- ❏ Whole grain muffin or loaf

Donuts, chips, churros

- ❏ Air-popped popcorn
- ❏ Bagel
- ❏ Nuts
- ❏ Seeds
- ❏ Soft pretzel
- ❏ Soy nuts

Ice cream (premium)

- ❏ 100% fruit juice bar
- ❏ Frozen fudge bar
- ❏ Frozen grapes
- ❏ Lower fat ice cream
- ❏ Frozen yogurt
- ❏ Unsweetened applesauce with cottage cheese

Milkshake, soda

- ❏ Banana Nutty Shake*
- ❏ Fruit spritzer
- ❏ Fruit smoothie
- ❏ Pudding
- ❏ Sweet Strawberry Nectar*

*See recipe at the end
of this chapter.

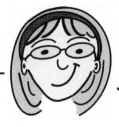

Did You Know?

You can help your child understand how much sugar is in a packaged food by teaching them to read labels. Here's how:

- **Find the amount.** Look on the side or back of a package for the Nutrition Facts panel. This box lists, among other things, the serving size and the amount (in grams) of "Total Sugars" in one serving.

- **Convert to a common measure.** Every 4 grams of sugar is the equivalent of 1 teaspoon of sugar. For example, a one-cup serving of a typical sugary cereal with 12 grams of Total Sugars is the same as sprinkling three teaspoons of sugar on it.

- **Adjust for reality.** Some brands use a ridiculously small serving size so the sugar content seems small. If your child's serving is different than the one listed in the box, multiply accordingly.

- **Find the source.** Look in the Ingredient list (it's right below the Nutrition Facts panel) to find the ingredients that contribute to the sugar content of the food.

As a rule of thumb, if sugar is listed among the top three ingredients, the food is likely high in sugar. Make sure these foods also have some fiber and protein to avoid blood sugar spikes.

Where Does Sugar Hide?

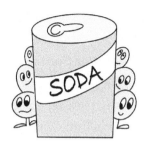

Sugar is naturally found in milk, fruit and other whole foods. But added sugars hide in many processed and packaged foods. In fact, most of the sugar in a child's diet isn't in plain sight in the sugar bowl. Rather, it's hiding in ultra-processed foods in the form of sucrose, high-fructose corn syrup, maple syrup, honey, agave and other forms of sugar.

For younger children, 2 to 8 years of age, the top two food sources of added sugars are sweetened beverages (fruit drinks, soda and teas) and sweet bakery products, followed by candy, ready-to-eat cereals and desserts. All together, these five food groups make up about two-thirds of a child's daily intake of added sugars. The trend is similar for older kids and teens, although sweetened tea and coffee drinks are more of a concern for this age group than desserts.[1] If you're like many parents, you may not be surprised sugar is hiding in processed and packaged foods marketed to your child. What may surprise you is where it's found. To learn more, see **Sugar Content of Common Foods for Kids** on page 159.[2]

A special caution about fruit drinks

In the U.S., the children's drink market is a multi-billion dollar industry. As you just learned, fruit drinks top the list as the most commonly consumed sugar-sweetened beverages. So, it's easy to see why marketers are serious about splashy labels, fun fruity images and health claims like "high in vitamin C" that hide the fact a drink is nothing more than sugar water with added vitamin C.

You would be forgiven if you think this is a confusing mess. After all, it's not unreasonable to rely on images and statements on the front of a package to decide whether a juice drink is healthful for your child. Many parents and caregivers do just that.

Yet, even the Food and Drug Administration, the agency that regulates the labels of fruit drinks and other foods, admits it's easy to be confused. In fact, under current regulations, marketers can be downright deceptive. For example, a fruit-flavored drink doesn't need to contain any fruit or fruit juice. Rather, the source of a drink's fruitiness could be nothing more than a flavoring (including an artificial one), and that's as far from real fruit juice as you can get.[3]

The FDA even warns consumers not to rely on a product's fanciful name, splashy package images or even its taste to determine if a fruit drink actually contains fruit or real fruit juice. Rather, you need to look at the Ingredient list. All packaged foods have one, and it's the only place a marketer is required to list all ingredients using common or usual names. Yes, regulations need to change, but in the meantime, you can rely on the Ingredient list to confirm your child is drinking real fruit juice and not just sugar water with a little flavoring. (You'll learn more in **Chapter 12: July – Label Reading Shortcuts**.)

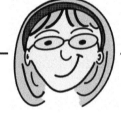

Did You Know?

Research supports the regular use of gum sweetened with xylitol or sorbitol to help prevent tooth decay.[4] Unlike sugar, these sweeteners aren't used by mouth bacteria to churn out cavity-producing acids, which is a distinct advantage over sugar-sweetened gums. The act of chewing also helps stimulate a healthy flow of saliva, which protects tooth enamel. When your child asks for a sweet, reach for a gum sweetened with one of these smile savers. It's a win-win situation: Less sugar and a healthier smile.

Sugar Content of Common Foods for Kids	
Food	**Amount of Sugar**
Yogurt, fruit, 1 cup	10½ teaspoons*
Soda, 12 ounces	10 teaspoons
Sports drink, 20 ounces	9 teaspoons
Yogurt, frozen, 1 cup	8¼ teaspoon
Fruit punch drink, 1 cup	7 teaspoons
100% Fruit juice, 1 cup	6 teaspoons*
Coconut, sweetened, 2 ounces	6 teaspoons*
Gelatin, flavored, ½ cup	5 teaspoons
Honey, 1 tablespoon	4¼ teaspoons*†
Pudding, ½ cup	4¼ teaspoons
Yogurt, plain, 1 cup	4¼ teaspoons*
Chocolate, 1 ounce	4 teaspoons
Cereal, sweetened, 1 cup	4 teaspoons
Ice cream, ½ cup	4 teaspoons
Milk, 1 cup	3 teaspoons*
Donut, cake type, 1 each	3¼ teaspoons
Yogurt, Greek, plain, 1 cup	2¼ teaspoons*
Figs, 1 each	1 teaspoon*
Jam, 1 teaspoon	1 teaspoon
Ketchup, 1 tablespoon	1 teaspoon
Chewing gum, 1 stick	½ teaspoon

*Predominately naturally occurring sugar.
†Also used as an added sugar in packaged and processed foods.
Source: USDA FoodData Central database (https://fdc.nal.usda.gov).

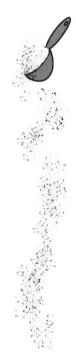

The Many Names of Sugar

The sugar in foods can hide behind a wide variety of names. To spot the most common sugar-based ingredients in packaged foods, simply look for the letters "ose" at the end of an ingredient's name such as dextrose, fructose, lactose, maltose, glucose, galactose and sucrose, just to name a few.

Other common names for sugary ingredients typically used to sweeten foods include barley malt syrup, brown rice syrup, brown sugar, corn syrup, high-fructose corn syrup, honey, maple syrup, molasses, raw sugar, sorbitol, sugar alcohols (lactitol, mannitol and others), syrup and turbinado sugar.

Caution: Energy Drain Ahead

To be sure, sugar-rich foods can provide a burst of quick energy, but the sharp energy drain that tends to follow can sap your child's ability to maintain focus and concentrate. For staying power in the classroom, choose foods rich in complex carbohydrates, such as whole grains. These foods are absorbed more slowly, providing a steady source of fuel to keep active brains focused throughout the school day. What's more, these foods are likely to be more nutrient dense, delivering their slow carbs along with other nourishing vitamins, minerals and fiber.

Parent Pearl

Replace soda with a fruit spritzer.
To satisfy my daughter's love for a sweet, fizzy drink, I serve up a fruit spritzer. It's a healthier alternative to soda and so easy to make. I simply add a dash of carbonated water to her favorite fruit juice. For extra flair, I top it off with a slice of lemon or orange.

A caveat about soda

Neither diet sodas nor regular sodas are a good choice for children (or adults for that matter). Regular sodas provide "empty calories" and contain nothing more than sugar (approximately 10 teaspoons per 12-ounce can), water, food coloring and flavor. While diet sodas do not contain calories, they fail to provide any nutritional value. Better choices are water, milk and fruit juice (in moderation).

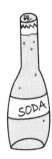

Excess sugar and its effects on learning

Diets loaded with sugar and fat, yet lacking in essential fatty acids, may lower the level of a critical bioactive compound in the brain involved in learning and memory. It's called brain-derived neurotropic factor (BDNF), and it's responsible for the development of new brain tissue and, therefore, for the formation of new memories.

Emerging research in laboratory rats reveals a direct link between the level of BDNF in the brain and the ability to learn spatial and memory tasks. What's more, when the laboratory rats were fed a diet high in sugar and fat, it only took two months to significantly reduce the level of BDNF in the brain and impact the animal's ability to perform spatial and memory tasks. More studies are needed to confirm a similar action in humans, but in the meantime, the findings add to the growing body of research that supports the brain benefits of avoiding excess sugar.[5]

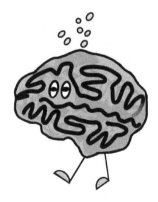

The Low Down on Sugar Substitutes

If you want to cut down on your child's sugar intake, you may be wondering about some of the sugar substitutes and sugar alternatives available in the marketplace.

Currently, the U.S. Food and Drug Administration (FDA) has approved seven sugar substitutes for use in foods sold in the United States: acesulfame potassium, aspartame, monk fruit, neotame, saccharin, stevia and sucralose.[6] The safety data for each of these sweeteners has been reviewed by national regulatory agencies, including the FDA, and by international health authorities, including the World Health Organization (WHO). The current consensus is each sweetener appears to be safe for use by all consumers, including children. Although, we recommend you choose natural ones like monk fruit and stevia rather than artificial ones.

Acesulfame potassium

Acesulfame potassium is an artificial sweetener that's heat stable, so it can be used in cooking and baking. It's often used in combination with other sweeteners such as saccharin in carbonated low-calorie beverages and other products. It's also available as a tabletop sweetener. This sugar substitute is about 200 times sweeter than white sugar (sucrose).

Aspartame

Aspartame is an artificial sweetener that's about 160 to 220 times sweeter than white sugar. It's not considered a "non-caloric" sweetener since it's broken down in the digestive tract into components that are absorbed and metabolized. However, because it's so sweet, just a small amount is needed to impart a big sweet taste. So, for all intents and purposes, the calories it provides are negligible. A word of caution: Children with the rare genetic disorder called phenylketonuria or PKU must avoid this sweetener as they are unable to break it down. (The color of individual packets is typically blue.)

Monk fruit

Also known as luo han guo, this natural sweetener is a fruit extract that's about 150 to 300 times sweeter than white sugar. It's used as a tabletop sweetener, a food ingredient and a component of other sweetener blends. It may have an aftertaste at high levels. (The color of individual packets is typically orange.)

Neotame

Neotame is an artificial sweetener that has a powerfully intense sugary taste, approximately 7,000 to 13,000 times sweeter than white sugar.

Saccharin

Saccharin, the first artificial sweetener to market, is about 300 times sweeter than white sugar. It's found in many dietetic food and beverage products. (The color of individual packets is typically pink.)

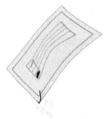

Stevia

Stevia is a plant-derived natural sweetener that's about 250 times sweeter than white sugar. (The color of individual packets is typically green.)

Sucralose

Sucralose is an artificial, non-caloric sweetener made from sugar. The body is unable to digest it, so it's excreted unchanged. It's about 600 times sweeter than white sugar. (The color of individual packets is typically yellow.)

Take home message

As a general rule, choose whole foods whenever possible. Rely on the natural sweetness of fruits and limit the intake of refined sweeteners. Again, if you do use sugar substitutes, we recommend you pass on the artificial ones and use natural ones like monk fruit or stevia.

Healthy Classroom Celebrations

With childhood obesity on the rise, more schools are encouraging parents to bring healthier foods for birthday and other celebrations during the school day. Here are a few options to consider for your child's next classroom celebration. Check with your child's teacher first, but we think the healthier options will be welcomed. Who knows, you just may start a trend.

Food items:

☐ Angel food cake, strawberries and whipped cream
☐ Carrot muffins (with just enough frosting for a smiley face)
☐ Fruit kabobs
☐ Pizza with 100% juice boxes
☐ Popcorn
☐ Pudding
☐ Snap peas or other veggies with a tasty dip
☐ Watermelon
☐ Yogurt parfait (see recipe on page 169)

Non-food items:

☐ A special book to read aloud and then donate to the class library
☐ Erasers
☐ Pencils
☐ Stickers
☐ Washable tattoos

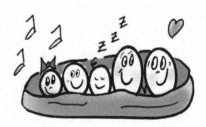

Tips to Reduce Refined Sugar

If you need inspiration for ways to help cut refined sugar in your child's diet, check out the tips below.

- ❑ **Go natural.** Buy fresh fruits or fruits packed in water or juice, rather than packed in light or heavy syrup.

- ❑ **Buy fewer sugary foods.** Fewer prepared baked goods, candies, sweet desserts, soft drinks and fruit-flavored drinks means less temptation.

- ❑ **Reduce the sugar in foods you prepare at home.** Out of sight, out of mind. Start by reducing sugar gradually until you've reduced it by one-third or more.

- ❑ **Add less sugar.** Have your child add less sugar to cereal. It's easy to get used to using half as much.

- ❑ **Eat regular meals.** Offer meals and snacks throughout the day to help curb your child's sweet tooth. Hunger is a sure-fire way to tempt your child to eat a sugary snack.

- ❑ **Read labels.** If any sugar is listed first on the ingredient list, use discretion or look for another option.

- ❑ **Add a pinch of salt.** It will enhance a food's natural sweetness.

- ❑ **Buy breakfast cereals without added sugars.** Your child will consume less sugar even with a sprinkle of their own sugar on top. (Some cereals are more like a dessert with over 3 teaspoons of sugar per serving, and kids often don't stop at one serving).

- ❑ **Train taste buds to be accustomed to less.** By avoiding sugary foods for as little as a week, your child will be able to taste the natural sweetness in foods and be less tempted by sugary foods.

- ❑ **Keep within the empty-calorie limit and use wisely** (see page 287). These calories are limited, so choose foods that really count. For most kids, this means desserts. Don't waste these calories on sodas and sugary breakfast cereals.

- ❑ **Experiment with spices.** Cinnamon, cardamom, coriander, nutmeg, ginger and other spices enhance flavor without sugar.

- ❑ **Serve sweet foods warm.** Heat enhances sweetness.

Banana Nutty Shake

This nutritious shake only needs four ingredients for a flavor burst that will have your child begging for more!

Ingredients

1 banana, frozen and broken into chunks
1 cup non-fat or low-fat milk
2 teaspoons honey
1 handful walnuts (about 6 halves)

Directions

1. In a blender, add banana, milk and honey.
2. Blend till smooth, about 45 seconds.
3. Add walnuts and blend for a few additional seconds.
4. Serve and enjoy!

Makes 2 servings (1 cup per serving)

164 **Calories** | 4g **Fat** | 26g **Carbs** | 6g **Protein**

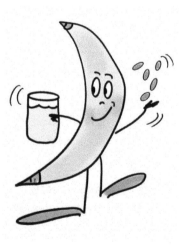

Blueberry Mini Muffins

This tasty breakfast addition or snack treat combines the antioxidant power of blueberries with hearty whole grain goodness and flaxseed, a natural source of omega-3 fats.

Ingredients

½ cup vanilla soymilk
½ cup apple juice concentrate
¼ cup canola oil
1 egg
1 cup whole wheat flour
1 cup oats
¼ cup milled flaxseed

⅓ cup sugar
3 teaspoons baking powder
½ teaspoon salt
1 cup blueberries
¼ cup walnut, chopped

Directions

1. Preheat oven to 400 degrees.

2. Grease bottoms of 36 mini-muffin cups or line with paper baking cups.

3. In a bowl, beat soymilk, apple juice concentrate, oil and egg. Stir in flour, oats, flaxseed, sugar, baking powder and salt until flour is moistened, but batter is lumpy. Fold in blueberries and nuts.

4. Divide batter evenly among muffin cups.

5. Bake for 15 minutes or until golden brown.

6. Remove immediately from pan to cool.

7. Serve and enjoy!

Freeze some muffins for school lunches. Add a frozen muffin to the lunch box during morning prep, and it will be perfectly thawed by lunch time.

Makes 36 servings (one muffin per serving)

55 **Calories** | 2g **Fat** | 8g **Carbs** | 1g **Protein**

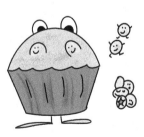

Brainy Banana Bread

This tasty bread is sure to please even your most finicky critic.

Ingredients

½ cup sugar
¼ cup butter, softened
1 egg
2 bananas, mashed
¼ cup milk
¾ cup whole wheat flour
½ cup white flour

1 teaspoon vanilla
1 teaspoon cinnamon
4 tablespoons milled flaxseed
½ teaspoon baking soda
½ teaspoon salt
½ cup walnuts, chopped

Directions

1. Preheat oven to 350 degrees.
2. In a bowl, combine sugar and butter; mix well. Add egg, bananas, milk and flour; blend well.
3. Stir in remaining ingredients, except nuts, until just moistened.
4. Add nuts, but save a few for later.
5. Pour batter into a greased 8½x4½x2½-inch loaf pan.
6. Sprinkle top with remaining nuts. Bake for about 60 minutes or until a wooden toothpick inserted in the center comes out clean. Remove from pan to cool.
7. Cut into slices, serve and enjoy!

Makes 16 serving (1 slice per serving)

120 **Calories** ∣ 4g **Fat** ∣ 18g **Carbs** ∣ 3g **Protein**

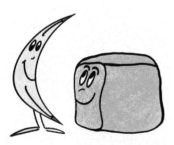

Fruity Yogurt Parfait

This colorful snack or dessert is a feast for the eyes and a rich source of protein and calcium.

Ingredients

6 ounces vanilla yogurt, or flavor of your choice

¼ cup granola

½ cup strawberries, or other favorite fruit, cut into slices

Directions

1. In a clear cup, alternate layers of yogurt, granola and strawberries.

2. Add a parasol for a colorful touch.

3. Serve and enjoy!

Makes 2 servings (¾ cup per serving)

155 **Calories** | 3g **Fat** | 28g **Carbs** | 4g **Protein**

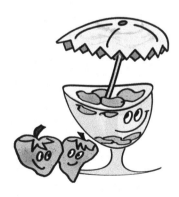

Going Coconuts for Pineapple Cake

When you have this tasty cake in the oven, don't be surprised if your little darling calls out, "Smells good, Mom!" You'll be pleased the recipe calls for no added sugars.

Ingredients

Wet ingredients

½ cup chopped apricots, fresh or well-drained (about 6 medium)

¾ cup crushed pineapple, well-drained

½ cup apple juice concentrate

1 cup low-fat milk

2 eggs

¼ cup canola oil

1 teaspoon vanilla extract

Dry ingredients

2 cups whole wheat flour

⅓ cup unbleached white flour

1 teaspoon baking soda

3 teaspoons baking powder

2 teaspoons cinnamon

⅓ cup coconut, flaked

Optional (add with coconut)

8 apricots, dried, chopped

¼ cup walnuts, chopped

4 tablespoons milled flaxseed

Directions

1. Preheat oven to 350 degrees.

2. In a blender or food processor, add all wet ingredients and puree until smooth.

3. Place mixture in a large bowl and add the dry ingredients (except coconut). Beat well. Stir in coconut (and any optional ingredients).

4. Coat an 8x8-inch baking pan with vegetable spray and then pour in batter.

5. Bake for about 45 to 50 minutes or until an inserted toothpick comes out clean. Cool before cutting into slices.

6. Serve and enjoy!

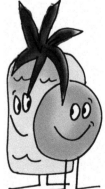

Makes 16 servings (1 slice per serving)

110 **Calories** | 6g **Fat** | 11g **Carbs** | 3g **Protein**

Sweet Strawberry Nectar

Talk about a winner. This fruit smoothie packs both flavor and nutrition, yet is oh-so-easy to whip up.

Ingredients

1 cup vanilla soymilk

5-6 strawberries, frozen

2 teaspoons whipped cream (optional)

Directions

1. In a blender, add soymilk and strawberries.

2. Blend until smooth, about 45 seconds.

3. Pour into cups, and if desired add a touch of whipped cream.

4. Serve and enjoy!

Consider buying a big bag of frozen strawberries, blueberries, blackberries or other berries, so you have plenty on hand.

Makes 2 servings (¾ cup per serving)

75 **Calories** | 1g **Fat** | 13g **Carbs** | 3g **Protein**

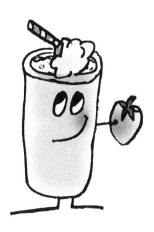

Yummy Crumbly Crisp

This delicious crisp is a snap to make.

Ingredients

⅓ cup butter, softened
½ cup brown sugar
1 teaspoon vanilla
½ cup flour
½ cup oats
¼ cup walnuts, chopped
6 cups sliced peaches (about 6 medium)*

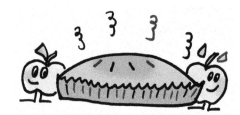

Directions

1. Preheat oven to 375 degrees. Grease 11½x8x2-inch pan.
2. In a bowl, combine butter, brown sugar and vanilla. Add flour and oats. Mix well.
3. Stir in walnuts.
4. Place fruit in pan and sprinkle oat mixture over top.
5. Bake for about 30 minutes or until topping is golden brown.
6. Serve warm and enjoy! If desired, add a dab of fresh whipped cream.

Makes 9 servings

200 **Calories** | 8g **Fat** | 28g **Carbs** | 3g **Protein**

*Alternative: Use other fruits or a combination of fruits. Tasty combos include apples, nectarines and blueberries or pears and raspberries. Use your imagination and have fun creating.

This Month's Smart Goal

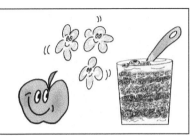

I will help my child brainstorm
a healthier substitute for one of their
frequent junk food choices this month.

This Month's Extra Credit

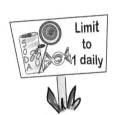

I will help my child limit sweets to once daily.

To monitor your daily progress toward your goals, use the **My Smart Tracker** forms in **Chapter 14: Go for the Goal.**

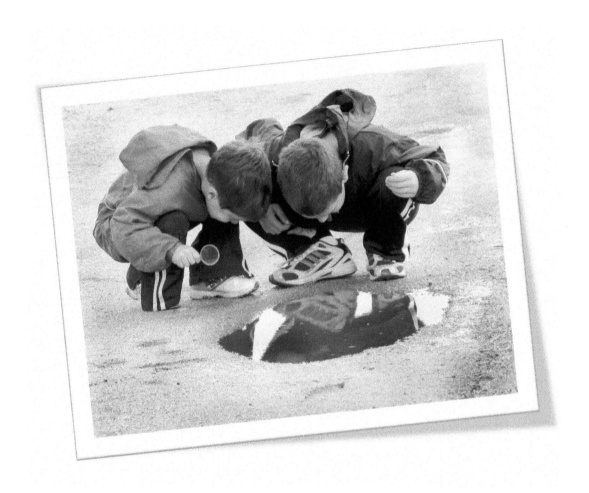

The mind that opens to a new idea
never returns to its original size.
– Albert Einstein

Chapter 10

May – New Foods for Curious Minds

Introducing your child to new, healthy foods is a perfect way to stimulate an active mind while nourishing the brain. Trouble is, most kids turn their noses up at the mere mention of a food that's packed with brain-building nutrition for no other reason than it's unfamiliar.

If your child is a picky eater, don't despair. Kids are actually hard-wired to avoid new foods.[1] Researchers call this "food neophobia" or a fear of new foods. They believe it's a genetic trait that may have developed to help us avoid unfamiliar foods that could be poisonous.

For cavemen who relied on hunting and gathering for food, this initial aversion to unfamiliar foods was a good thing. Today, however, our foraging is typically limited to trips to the local supermarket or farmer's market where foods are generally safe. So, in today's world, food neophobia actually works against us because it can limit the variety of fruits, vegetables and other nutrient-dense foods we eat that support brain health.

You can help your child overcome food neophobia by rethinking how you introduce new foods. Remember, kids are more likely to eat foods that are familiar. So, your goal is to make a food more familiar. To do this, you'll want to offer a new food often and in a variety of interesting ways. Regular exposure and variety are the perfect combination to help ease any fear of new foods and expand the variety of nutritious foods your child will want to try. Be creative and stick with it. You'll soon see little fingers eager to try the newly familiar (and nutritious) foods.

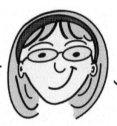

Did You Know?

In one review of the scientific literature, university researchers ranked the effectiveness of things we often do to entice kids to eat more vegetables. This includes teaching kids about good nutrition, cooking and other fun educational activities, making dishes look more appealing such as serving in a colorful bowl, and sneaking veggies into meals such as in purees. While many of these techniques work, one method stands out as best.

"Which one?" you might ask. The very best way to help young children eat more vegetables is to simply give them plenty of chances to taste them. How many times do you keep offering a new vegetable before a child will give it the thumbs up? The researchers say at least 8 to 10 times.[2]

Smart Moves for More Variety

Here are 12 key strategies you can start using right now to help introduce your child to new food experiences. Choose one to start and then build from there. You'll soon be rewarded with a child who enjoys a wider variety of nutritious foods to better fuel their active brain.

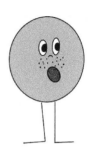

1 **Stock your home with more healthy foods.** Few habits will have more impact on what your child eats at home than your efforts to bring more healthy foods into your home, including fruits and vegetables.

2 **Make healthy choices ready-to-serve.** Don't underestimate the value of preparing foods to be ready when your child is looking for a snack. For example, wash grapes, cut them into small bunches and place them in a bowl in the fridge. In this way, you make the healthy choice the easiest one. And, since little or no preparation is required on your child's part, it's likely to be the first choice.

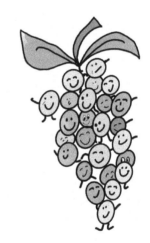

3 **Limit junk food at home.** The easiest way to curtail your child's intake of junk food at home is to avoid bringing it into your kitchen.

4 **Limit goodies to one serving at a time.** If you choose to bring a few not-so-nutritious "goodies" into your home, serve them up in single-serving portions to discourage overeating. This is especially important when you purchase oversized items typically sold at warehouse club stores. The larger sizes may be friendly on your budget, but they can encourage overeating. Serve one serving, then put the rest away in the pantry, fridge or freezer. Leaving the container in plain view tends to encourage a second or third helping.

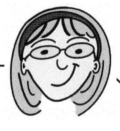

Did You Know?

Most people tend to eat the same foods day in and day out. Makes sense since we're creatures of habit, but it can also limit the variety of foods your child eats and the chance to consume a wider range of nutrients.

One way to add more variety to your child's diet is with whole grains. Has your child tried barley, bran, brown rice, bulgur, cornmeal, kasha, oat bran, quinoa, wheat germ, whole wheat or another whole grain? All are excellent sources of fiber with its nourishing benefits like helping curb hunger, promote regularity and balance healthy gut bacteria, just to name a few. Why not make a trip to a local store that features these grains in bulk bins and try one? Who knows, you may stumble on a healthy winner.

5 **Encourage your kids to ask, "Where's the fruit or veggie?" at every meal.** Whether it's fresh, frozen, canned or juice, it all counts. If it's missing, ask what can be added to complete the meal. This habit helps your kids become comfortable with the notion that a complete meal includes at least one fruit or vegetable like banana slices on morning cereal, a crisp apple at lunch or steamed carrots at dinner.

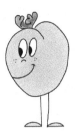

6 **Model healthy eating habits.** Be adventurous yourself about trying new foods. Kids notice more than you may think and are likely to try foods that their parents or older siblings enjoy.

7 **Don't be fooled by junk foods masquerading as healthy choices.** Foods with no nutritional value are nothing more than junk food regardless of their food group. For example, a trendy new breakfast cereal may be loaded with sugar and have a nutritional profile more like a candy bar. If these types of foods are on your kid's must-have list, treat them like any other junk food—an occasional choice rather than a daily staple.

8 **Try different textures.** Don't forget that the texture of food is especially important for children, so before giving up on introducing a new food, experiment with different textures. Your little one may pass on crisp apple slices but gobble up applesauce with a smile.

> **Parent Pearl**
>
> **Homework is a breeze in our house with two simple rules.** First, I encourage the kids to tackle the tough stuff when their confidence is high, then they can breeze through easier assignments later. We also have a "stick-with-it" rule: The shortest amount of time to spend on a tough subject before switching gears.

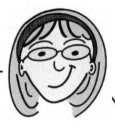

Did You Know?

Growing your own vegetables is easier than you may think when you use the square foot gardening techniques inspired by Mel Bartholomew. Thanks to a little engineering genius, he created a simple, yet elegant way to grow more in less space. Your home improvement store is sure to have all the basics to get started—planting box, seeds and soil mix.

Grab the kids and spend a few hours on a weekend afternoon mixing your soil and planting your seeds. Pick a spot where it's easy to water frequently. The kids will love watching those tiny seeds transform into ripe tomatoes, sugar snap peas, plump zucchini and other nutritious vegetables. What's more, in a few short weeks, you'll be rewarded with a bounty of vegetables worthy of your dinner table and kids who are eager to eat them. Need more inspiration to get started? Visit www.squarefootgardening.com.

9 **Don't make it a big deal.** If your child turns down new foods, don't stress. Keep offering them. It may take several attempts before your child acquires a taste for it. What's more, a little reverse psychology ("Excellent, more for me!") may be all that's needed for a change of mind.

10 **Add some fun.** Kids can be picky about the way a food looks, but adding some fun can help entice them. Draw a raisin smile on a bowl of oatmeal. Create a broccoli forest by standing broccoli florets in mashed potatoes. Let your creativity shine so you can introduce new foods in a fun way.

11 **Introduce new foods with old favorites.** The "halo" effect will help link the good thoughts and feelings about favorite foods to a new food served along with it. Introduce green beans sprinkled with your child's favorite nuts such as crunchy slivers of almonds. Introduce okra in a favorite vegetable soup. Introduce whole wheat pasta with a favorite marinara sauce. Introduce almond or soy butter by spreading it on a favorite cracker.

12 **Banish the "yucky" color syndrome.** If your child has proclaimed all foods of one color are "yucky," consider serving them with a favorite food of another color. Serve zucchini with melted cheese; celery with peanut butter; kiwi slices with a dollop of whipped cream.

> **Parent Pearl**
>
> **Once a month, we have breakfast for dinner.** I serve up the kids' favorites—cereal, toast and grapefruit; pancakes topped with maple syrup; or a tomato and cheese omelet. By switching things up, the kids learn to be creative and see that any healthy food choice is welcome at every meal.

This Month's Smart Goal

I will serve at least one new fruit, vegetable or whole grain food each week.

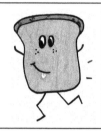

This Month's Extra Credit

I will start a "square foot" garden.

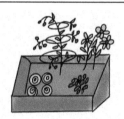

To monitor your daily progress toward your goals, use the **My Smart Tracker** forms in **Chapter 14: Go for the Goal.**

Part 5

Summer Fun

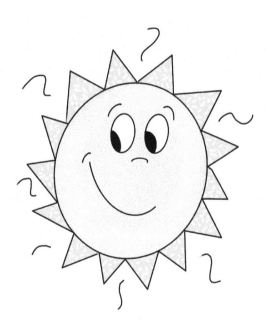

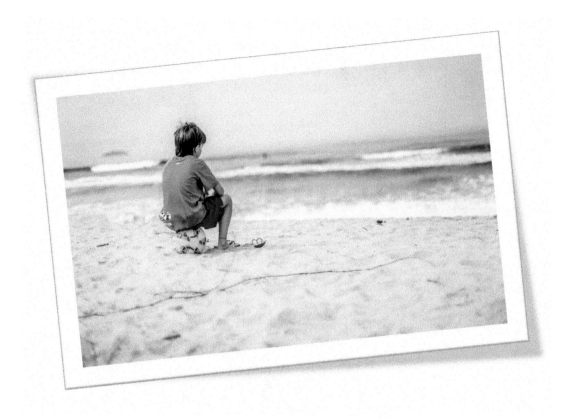

Water is the driving force of all nature.
— Leonardo da Vinci

Chapter 11

June – The Wonders of Water

It's time to welcome in the sunny days of summer, but as temperatures rise, so too does your child's need for fluid. Since staying well hydrated is essential for peak performance (both mental and physical), there's no better time to focus on helping your child consume an adequate intake of water. Yet, if you're like most people, you may be overlooking the importance of this versatile nutrient.

Not only is water essential to digest food, but it's needed for lymph, the immune system fluid that helps ward off illness. Water also transports nutrients throughout the body, helps get rid of excess heat through sweat and removes toxic byproducts from the body.

What's more, water is critical for the brain to function properly. In fact, the majority of the brain is made up of water. And, it's no coincidence more than 80% of the brain region used for learning and memory (the hippocampus) is water.[1] In other words, optimal mental function depends on optimal hydration.

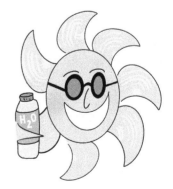

How Much Water Is Enough?

When you think of your child's water intake, you may think of drinking water or other beverages. Many parents do. Yet, foods like fruits and vegetables, soups, yogurts and the like also contribute to your child's daily water intake.

For this reason, nutrition experts often talk about "total water intake." That is, the amount your child consumes every day from both foods (about 25%) and beverages (about 75%). For example, the National Academy of Medicine (formerly known as the Institute of Medicine) recommends young girls and boys, age 4 to 8 years, get about 7 cups of total water per day (5 cups from drinking water and other beverages). Older girls and boys, age 9 to 13 years, need a bit more, about 9 to 10 cups of total water per day with most of it (7 to 8 cups) from drinking water or other beverages.[2]

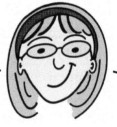

Did You Know?

While summer typically signals a break from the traditional classroom setting, it still offers many learning opportunities from taking nature hikes to visiting museums, libraries or other cultural centers. In fact, any outing can be a time to grow brain cells and make new connections. Be sure to take full advantage of these activities, especially ones that help polish math skills. Research shows the first two to four months of a new school year are devoted to relearning previous material. Sadly, math skills are especially prone to decline.[3] To keep skills sharp over the summer months, consider developing a routine so that your child learns something new every day.

Take a practical approach

While the National Academy of Medicine's recommended water guidelines are good advice, they're not the most practical. A more practical approach is to encourage your child to be a scientist. Before flushing, ask your child to take a quick peek at the color of their urine in the toilet bowl. If it's dark like the color of apple juice, it's likely a sign of dehydration, and they need to drink more water. If it's only slightly yellow like the color of lemonade, then your child is likely well hydrated. Other signs of dehydration are smelly urine or the ability to produce only a small amount of it.

Exceptions to the rule

There are a few exceptions to these urine color and smell rules. For example, if your child recently took a multivitamin, the results may be skewed. Why? Many multivitamins contain riboflavin, a B vitamin that can turn urine bright yellow. Likewise, eating beets will produce urine with a reddish hue.

In addition, some people who eat asparagus say they have very smelly urine. It's normal and appears to depend on their genetic makeup. Researchers point to variations in genes associated with smell (olfactory receptor genes), which can make some people especially good at sniffing out asparagus metabolites in urine. In other words, these people have a more finely tuned sense of smell that's better at detecting the stinky stuff.[4]

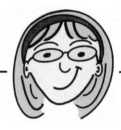

Did You Know?

Dehydration is the most preventable sports injury. Consider weighing your child before and after a sports event. For every pound lost, make sure your child drinks at least 16 ounces (2 cups) of water to adequately replenish fluid lost in sweat.

Drink Up to Avoid Sports Injury

Getting enough water is critical if you have a sporty child. The combination of exertion and heat can cause a decrease in performance, but more importantly, it can be harmful to your child's overall health. In fact, you might say proper hydration is your child's secret weapon to be their best self at whatever activity they choose.

Not only does proper hydration help delay fatigue, it helps maintain mental sharpness and physical performance (think agility and reaction time), and it helps reduce stress on the heart. Proper hydration also helps your child regulate their body heat, which can help prevent heat-related illnesses. And, it helps speed up recovery so your child can continue to enjoy being active.

You can easily help your active child stay properly hydrated by following a few guidelines:

- Think of fluids as part of your child's essential safety equipment.
- Bring the right kinds of fluids to practices and competitions.
- Drink before, during and after activity.
- Check hydration status by monitoring the color of urine.

Parent Pearl

I look for fun ways to practice math skills with my kids during our regular routine. We track and chart the daily temperature. When driving, I give the kids math challenges or ask them to read a map. When shopping, I ask them how much change we should get back. It's a great way to keep their skills sharp.

Sports Drinks: Best & Worst

Hands down, the best drink for everyday hydration is water. However, if your child is exercising or playing a competitive sport that lasts more than one hour, then some of the commercial electrolyte drink options may be a better bet. These beverages help replenish electrolytes, such as sodium and potassium, and vitamins, such as the B vitamins, that are lost in excess sweat or are needed in greater amounts.

Taste counts

If your child just doesn't like water, try offering a lightly flavored beverage. Research suggests that the added flavor may encourage your child to drink more and stay better hydrated.

Keep it cool

If your child participates in activities performed in hot weather, try offering cold beverages. This can help reduce their core body temperature and, thus, improve their performance in the heat.[5]

Pass on soft drinks

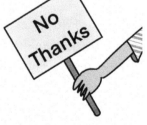

Soft drinks are nothing more than liquid sugar that fill your child's diet with empty calories. Unfortunately, kids (and teens) are now drinking soda with alarming frequency. In fact, almost two-thirds of children (62%) and teens (61%) report drinking soda or other sugar-sweetened beverages like sweetened fruit juices, nectars, sports drinks and energy drinks on any given day, according to a 2011-2016 NHANES national nutrition survey.[6] In practical terms, this means an average daily intake of about 14 ounces for young children (5 to 11 years of age) and 20 ounces for teens.

Is Tap Water So Terrible?

Many people choose bottle water because they believe it's purer than tap water; others claim taste and convenience are most important. However, one of the most common reasons people turn the tap off and reach for the bottle is the perception that bottled water is a safer option.

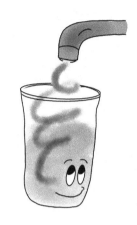

To better understand how accurate this perception is, it helps to know how the two products are regulated. Bottled water is considered a food, so it's regulated by the U.S. Food and Drug Administration (FDA). Tap water, by contrast, is regulated by the U.S. Environmental Protection Agency (EPA).

Both bottled and tap varieties of water may contain contaminants such as bacteria, arsenic, lead or other heavy metals, or pesticides, but both also undergo testing to confirm contamination, if any, is low enough to be considered safe. Most healthy adults can tolerate exposure to trace amounts of these contaminants. Children and other groups, however, may be sensitive to even low levels of contaminants. To learn more about the purity of the tap water in your area, visit the EPA's website at www.epa.gov/ground-water-and-drinking-water.

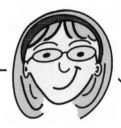

Did You Know?

Sodas and fruit drinks can overload your child's diet with empty calories. Consider the following healthful alternatives at meals: milk or fruit juice (perhaps mixed with sparkling water). Between meals, however, have your child reach for thirst-quenching water. Don't forget to be a role model: When your child sees you drinking water, they're likely to ask for it too.

A Word About Single-Use Plastic Water Bottles

You don't need headline news to know single-use plastic water bottles are among the most destructive products on the planet. Rather, you need only look at the waste filling our oceans, lakes and rivers, and piling up on land. Here's a not-so-fun fact: Single-use plastics account for almost half of all plastic pollution.[7]

The reason may seem obvious: By design, a single-use plastic product like a water bottle is supposed to be used only once and then discarded, leaving an unsightly mess that piles up fast. According to EarthDay.org, Americans purchase about 50 billion water bottles per year. That's an average of about 13 bottles per month for every person in the United States.[8]

What's less obvious is the serious impact you can make when your child switches to a reusable stainless steel water bottle. Not only is it better for their body, but also for the planet. Plus, imagine the money you'll save. But, if your child does drink water from plastic bottles, here are a few basics for safer use:

1 **Sniff and taste.** If there's any hint of plastic odor or taste in your water, don't drink it.

2 **Keep bottled water away from heat.** This helps prevent chemicals in the plastic from leaching into the water.

3 **Don't reuse bottles intended for single use.** They are a potential breeding ground for harmful bacteria.

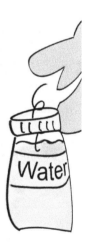

Cost-Saving Filter Options

If you like the taste and quality of bottled water, but want more bang for your buck, consider the cost-saving value of a high-quality water filter.

Water purified with these products generally costs less than buying bottled water, up to 90% less by some estimates.

Experts report you can feel confident about the water quality provided by reputable brand name home filtration systems. However, a word to the wise: Make sure that you follow the manufacturer's instructions. Without proper maintenance, it's possible bacteria or other contaminants can build up in these filtration systems.

Parent Pearl

When my daughter says, "I'm hungry, mommy," I always offer water first. Since much of hunger is actually thirst, it's an easy way to help make sure she stays properly hydrated.

The Caffeine Scoop

Caffeine increases the body's ability to expel water. This diuretic effect can lead to dehydration in your child. For this reason, kids should limit their caffeine intake. In fact, there's really no need to introduce caffeinated foods or beverages into your child's diet. We suggest you avoid them, but as a general rule of thumb, aim to limit your child's caffeine intake to no more than 2.5 milligrams of caffeine per kilogram body weight.[9] In practical terms, this means about 1 milligram of caffeine per pound of body weight. For more specific guidelines, use the chart below.

Upper Limit for Daily Caffeine Intake	
Body Weight	**Caffeine Amount**
30 lbs	34 milligrams
40 lbs	45 milligrams
50 lbs	57 milligrams
60 lbs	68 milligrams
70 lbs	80 milligrams
80 lbs	91 milligrams
90 lbs	102 milligrams
100 lbs	114 milligrams
110 lbs	125 milligrams
120 lbs	136 milligrams
130 lbs	148 milligrams
Source: Health Canada. Available at: www.canada.ca/en/health-canada.	

Where Does Caffeine Hide?

Coffee isn't the only food with caffeine. In fact, caffeine shows up in a wide variety of foods that may be a part of your child's regular diet. Here are a few of the more common foods with hidden caffeine:

Food Group	Serving Size	Caffeine*
Coffee		
Regular, brewed	8 fl. oz.	120 mg
Ready-to-drink (bottled or canned)	8 fl. oz.	100 mg
Specialty (latte, mocha, cappuccino, Americano)	8 fl. oz.	95 mg
Espresso (single shot)	1 fl. oz.	60 mg
Carbonated Soft Drinks		
All types (cola, citrus & other flavors)	12 fl. oz.	55 mg
Tea		
Tea, yerba mate (brewed)	8 fl. oz.	125 mg
Tea, black (brewed)	8 fl. oz.	45 mg
Tea, instant powder	8 fl. oz.	30 mg
Tea, ready-to-drink, bottled	8 fl. oz.	25 mg
Tea, green (brewed)	8 fl. oz.	25 mg
Tea, white (brewed)	8 fl. oz.	15 mg
Energy Drinks/Shots		
Energy drinks	8 fl. oz.	180 mg
Energy shots	1 fl. oz.	65 mg
Chocolate Foods and Beverages		
Chocolate bar, sweet/dark	1 bar (1.45 oz.)	25 mg
Chocolate milk, hot cocoa	8 fl. oz.	about 5 mg
Chocolate ice cream, frozen yogurt, flavored yogurt	1 cup (135 grams)	about 5 mg

* Amounts are approximate; mg indicates milligrams.
Source: USDA FoodData Central. Available at: https://fdc.nal.usda.gov.

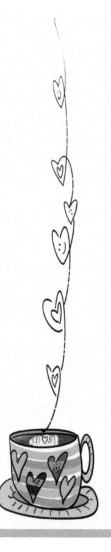

Eight Brain Boosters for Summer Days

If you need inspiration for fun activities to challenge your child's mental skills during the summer months, read on for eight sure-to-please options to consider:

1 **Read, read and read some more.** If you are taking a vacation or visiting a new city or other destination, research the trip ahead of time with your child. It's sure to build excitement and anticipation. Whether your plans include crossing the Panama Canal, hiking the trails at Yosemite or simply catching the tadpoles at the local park, reading about and researching the experience together ahead of time will make it come alive.

2 **Word morph.** Pick a three-letter word and change one letter at a time. Take turns and see how many different words you can come up with. Dog to dig to big to rig to rip to tip. You get the idea.

3 **Encourage letter writing and drawing.** To keep your child's writing skills sharp and the communication lines open, encourage letter writing to friends and relatives during the summer months. Scan the letters to a digital file before sending for a great keepsake. You can also scan artwork and other well-done school projects to enjoy for years to come.

Parent Pearl

I've become a scanning guru thanks to my daughter's love of drawing. I want to preserve her work, so when a new masterpiece is ready, I scan it right away and save a digital file. It's a great way to preserve these treasures to enjoy for years to come.

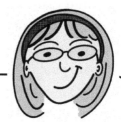

Did You Know?

One of the best resources for the freshest fruits and vegetables for your table is your community's farmers market. It's a win-win situation. You support your local farmers, and they deliver seasonal produce at the peak of nutrition. To find a list of farmers markets near you, visit the Local Harvest website at www.localharvest.org.

4 **The newspaper sleuth.** Make a list of age-appropriate questions with answers that can be found in the daily newspaper.

5 **Take an alphabet walk.** Enjoy a walk together and take turns finding objects in the order of the alphabet: ant, bee, concrete, dirt and so on.

6 **Zany alliterations.** Molly Magee makes marvelous mud pies. Consider starting with the letter A and then try the letter B. The wackier, the better.

7 **Fictionary.** Pick an obscure word from the dictionary and write down its meaning. Have others write a definition as well. Read out the various definitions. Award one point to the person who gets the answer correct, award one point to the person who made up a definition that fooled the others, and award one point to each person stumped by the person who chose the word.

8 **Visit the local library.** Take a trip to your local public library at least once a week. It's a community treasure that offers inexpensive access to a wide selection of books, enrichment programs and other resources. Your child can choose several books each week to read or have read to them.

Parent Pearl

On the first day of summer vacation, the kids and I brainstorm summer activities. We make a list of all the things we want to do during the break. We usually come up with at least 50 ideas. As we do them, we check them off. Now, I rarely hear the kids say, "I'm bored."

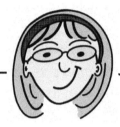

Did You Know?

If you're on snack duty for your child's sports team, choosing juicy orange slices, tangy cranberry juice and crunchy almonds will not only refuel the kids, but will provide added antioxidant protection.

This Month's Smart Goal

I will have my child track urine color and drink more water if the color resembles apple juice.

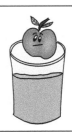

This Month's Extra Credit

I will make a summer "To Do" list with my family of activities that stimulate the mind, body and spirit.

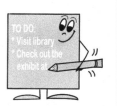

To monitor your daily progress toward your goals, use the **My Smart Tracker** forms in **Chapter 14: Go for the Goal.**

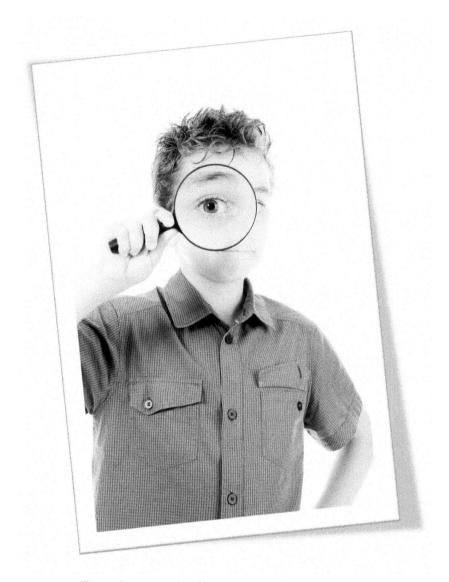

To eat is a necessity, but to eat intelligently is an art.
— La Rochefoucauld

Chapter 12

July – Label Reading Short Cuts

If you're like many parents, you're starved for time, which means grocery shopping often falls into the "I can't do it fast enough" category. Trouble is, the typical supermarket stocks almost 40,000 items, according to FMI, The Food Industry Association and their 2021 Supermarket Facts.[1] It's hard enough wrapping your mind around such a large number, let alone weave your way through the grocery aisles without feeling overwhelmed and frustrated.

With so many products competing for your time and attention, how do you quickly scan the shelves to find the best choices to feed your family? It's not easy, especially when it comes to ultra-processed foods with colorful packaging, splashy labels, and fun cartoon characters designed to appeal to kids.

You can simplify things by cutting through the marketing noise to get to information that matters. It starts with the nine label reading guidelines in this chapter. Apply these guidelines as you navigate your shopping cart down the grocery aisles, and you may be surprised at how quickly you'll become a pro at spotting healthier options.

Before we dive into each guideline, it's important to recognize that just about any food can fit into a healthy, balanced diet (unless a child has a medical issue that requires avoiding certain foods). In fact, banishing your child from occasionally eating a junk food with little or no nutritional value tends to backfire and makes the forbidden food even more appealing. A better choice is to use your label reading skills to separate packaged foods into two general categories: healthy, brain-building foods to enjoy regularly and less-than-nutritious foods to consume occasionally, if at all. Let's get started.

All facts, no puffery

Every time you pick up a new packaged food, make it a habit to look at the Nutrition Facts panel. With a few exceptions, it's on the side or back of a packaged food's label. (You'll find several examples in the pages that follow.) Why focus on this little gem? While a marketer can use colorful designs, fanciful images and health claims elsewhere on a label to entice you, they must follow precise rules required by the U.S. Food & Drug Administration (FDA) for the information they put in the Nutrition Facts panel. In other words, the Nutrition Facts panel is off limits to marketing puffery, making it one of the best tools you can use to evaluate a food's nutritional value.

The FDA not only regulates what kind of information can be included in the Nutrition Facts panel, but the agency also controls how it looks. No enticing bold colors, splashy copy or perky cartoon characters are permitted here.

In fact, compared to the marketing glitz elsewhere on food labels, the Nutrition Facts panel looks downright boring. But don't be fooled, it's filled with a wealth of information about what's in a food (and what's not). The trick is knowing what information to look for and how to use it to quickly spot brain-building foods to buy and brain-draining foods to leave on the shelf.

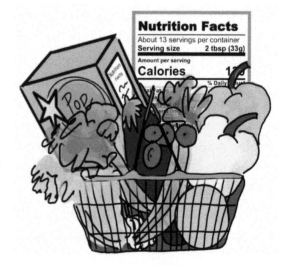

Guideline 1: A Serving Is Not a Portion

The serving size is the most important information in the Nutrition Facts panel. In fact, it's so important that the FDA requires food manufacturers to prominently display it at the top of the panel, making it especially easy to spot on packaged foods.

Why is the serving size so important? It's because it's the basis for all the other information in the Nutrition Facts panel. If you overlook it and jump right to scanning information about calories, fat and other nutrients, you'll likely overestimate or underestimate what your child is actually consuming.

The good news is, the FDA revised labeling regulations for the Nutrition Facts panel in 2016, including a big change in the requirements for the serving size. Now, a serving size must be based on the amount of a food a person is likely to eat in one sitting. Sounds reasonable, right?

Yet, previously, the serving size could be based on how much a person should consume rather than how much they're likely to consume. And, since all other nutrient information in the Nutrition Facts panel flows from the serving size, you can see why this label update is important.

Parent Pearl

When grocery shopping, I make sure to bring a list and to go when I'm not hungry. This helps prevent impulse buys. Shopping the outside aisles helps too. It's where dairy, produce, meats and other essentials are. In this way, I avoid many of the rows with packaged foods and focus on what I really need.

Potato Chips (Large Bag)

Look here for serving size. In the updated Nutrition Facts panel, it's big, bold and, for many foods, it better reflects portions people are more likely to eat.

Nutrition Facts

13 servings per container

Serving size   About 15 chips (28g)

Amount per serving

Calories   160

% Daily Value*

Total Fat 10g	**13%**
Saturated Fat 1.5g	**7%**
Trans Fat 0g	
Cholesterol 0mg	**0%**
Sodium 170mg	**7%**
Total Carbohydrate 15g	**6%**
Dietary Fiber 1g	**5%**
Total Sugars less than 1g	
Protein 2g	
Vitamin D 0mcg	0%
Calcium 10mg	0%
Iron 0.5mg	2%
Potassium 350mg	6%

Not a significant source of added sugars.

* The % Daily Value tells you how much a nutrient in a serving of food contributes to a daily diet. 2,000 calories a day is used for general nutrition advice.

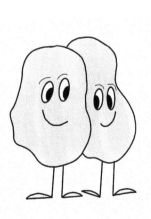

Servings, portions and handfuls

While the FDA increased serving sizes for some foods to better reflect real-world portions (double for some foods),[2] they missed the boat on others. Consider potato chips. A serving size remains 1 ounce (28 grams) whether the bag is jumbo-size or single-serving (see the example for a large bag of regular potato chips on the previous page). In practical terms, one serving is about 15 chips, about a handful. So, if your child's serving is closer to 30 chips, you'll need to double the amount of calories, fat, sodium and other nutrients listed in the Nutrition Facts panel to get an accurate measure of what your child is really eating.

How many servings are in your portion?

Here's a great exercise to visualize the difference between a typical portion and the serving size listed on a packaged food. The next time you offer your child potato chips, place them on your child's plate and then count them. Really, count them out. Now, check the label to see how close your portion is to the serving size listed in the Nutrition Facts panel. Is it closer to 15 chips (one serving), 30 chips (two servings) or more? For many people, a typical portion is two or more servings.

Guideline 2: Every Calorie Counts

Another key listing in the Nutrition Facts panel is calories per serving. Now that you're portion-size savvy, you can use the calorie information to accurately estimate how much a packaged food contributes to your child's daily needs.

Just how many calories does your child need to maintain a healthy body weight? It mostly depends on their age, sex and activity level. On average, younger kids, age 4 to 8 years, need between 1,200 and 2,000 calories per day to maintain a healthy body weight. Sedentary children—those who get less than 30 minutes of moderate physical activity on most days—have calorie needs on the low end of the range at about 1,200 to 1,400 calories per day. On the other hand, active kids—those who get the equivalent of a brisk three-mile walk every day—require a calorie intake on the high end of the range or about 1,400 to 2,000 calories per day.

The total calorie needs for older kids, age 9 to 13 years, are similar or higher, but the same activity rule applies: Active kids need more calories than their sedentary counterparts to maintain a healthy body weight. For more details, see **Recommended Daily Intake: Calories** on page 286.

Guideline 3: Wiggle, But Just A Little

Every diet deserves a little wiggle room for potato chips, cookies, and other less-than-nutritious foods. In fact, nutrition experts report there's no reason a healthy diet can't include a few of these foods with so-called "empty calories." The trick is to consume just enough to satisfy a craving, but not so much that filling up on them leads to excess weight gain or other health issues and prevents your child from eating enough nutrient-dense foods to fuel their body and brain.

What's the daily limit for empty calories?

According to the 2020-2025 Dietary Guidelines for Americans, a diet with up to 15% empty calories is still considered healthy. That's because these nutrition experts say we should be able to meet our nutritional needs when 85% of the foods we eat provide nutrient-dense calories. It's the same for kids. So, in practical terms, this means the amount of wiggle room for empty calories is only a few hundred calories per day. For more details, see **Recommended Daily "Empty Calorie" Limit** on page 287.

This may seem like plenty of calories for a splurge, but they can add up fast when your child is reaching for high-fat or sugar-laden processed foods. Consider

the potato chip example on page 206. Two servings of chips (320 calories) can easily meet or exceed a child's daily limit for empty calories. Whether the calories your child consumes are from nutrient-dense, healthy foods or empty calories, one fact remains true: Every calorie counts.

Guideline 4: Choose Fat like Goldilocks

For children, 4 years of age and older, tweens and teenagers, take the Goldilocks approach to total fat intake—not too little, not too much, but just the right amount for growing bodies and active brains. So, what's the "right" amount of fat for your child? According to the 2022-2025 Dietary Guidelines for Americans, a healthy fat intake for these ages is in the range of 25% to 35% of total daily calories.[3]

Simplify with the law of averages

How should you choose packaged foods to meet this guideline? The simplest way is to use the law of averages. Using grade-school math, you can calculate the percent calories from fat for any packaged food (more on this below). Armed with this information, you can choose more packaged foods that are lower in fat (no more than 35% fat calories) and fewer foods that are higher in fat. In this way, you can help keep your child's daily fat intake in the healthy range.

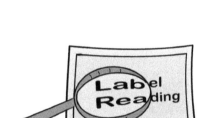

Where do you start?

The Nutrition Facts panel has all the information you need to calculate fat calories. Calories and Total Fat (in grams) is big and bold in the updated version, but percent calories from fat is gone, so a little light math is in order. To practice, check out the Nutrition Facts panel for a typical graham cracker on the next page.

Graham Crackers

Look here to calculate calories from fat:

3.5 grams fat
x 9 calories/gram
~ 32 fat calories

32 fat calories
÷ 130 total calories
X 100
~ 25% fat

Nutrition Facts

About 14 servings per container

Serving size   8 crackers (30g)
(1 serving = 2 full cracker sheets)

Amount per serving

Calories   130

	% Daily Value*
Total Fat 3.5g	4%
Saturated Fat 1g	5%
Trans Fat 0g	
Cholesterol 0mg	0%
Sodium 135mg	6%
Total Carbohydrate 23g	8%
Dietary Fiber 1g	4%
Total Sugars 7g	
Includes 7g Added Sugars	14%
Protein 2g	
Vitamin D 0mcg	0%
Calcium 20mg	0%
Iron 0.9mg	2%
Potassium 50mg	6%

* The % Daily Value tells you how much a nutrient in a serving of food contributes to a daily diet. 2,000 calories a day is used for general nutrition advice.

Ingredients: Unbleached Enriched Flour (Wheat Flour, Niacin, Iron, Thiamine Mononitrate, Riboflavin, Folic Acid), Whole Grain Wheat Flour, Sugar, **Canola Oil**, Molasses, **Palm Oil**, Leavening (Baking Soda and/or Calcium Phosphate), Salt.

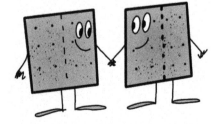

You'll see the serving size is two full cracker sheets, and each serving contains 130 calories and 3.5 grams of fat. By multiplying the grams of fat by 9 (one gram of fat contains 9 calories), you'll find a serving contains about 32 fat calories (rounded to the nearest whole calorie).

Next, divide fat calories by total calories and multiply by 100 to convert your answer to a percentage (32 fat calories/130 total calories x 100 = about 25%). In other words, graham crackers are 25% fat, making them a lower fat snack.

Using the Nutrition Facts panel to calculate a food's percent fat comes in handy when you're choosing packaged crackers and cookies, since these are favorite snack items for many kids.

Guideline 5: Avoid Brain-Draining Fats

The Nutrition Facts panel is also a wealth of information about the types of fats found in a packaged food. In fact, manufacturers of all packaged foods must now list both the amounts and types of fats in the Nutrition Facts panel. You'll find up to four types of fat listed, but only two are required (saturated and trans fats). You'll soon learn why this is important for your child's health. The two remaining types of fat (monounsaturated and polyunsaturated fats) may be listed, but aren't required unless a claim is made about them.

The troublesome duo

Of all types of fat, two are especially detrimental to growing brains: saturated fats and trans fats. Why? Diets high in saturated fats can lead to high blood cholesterol that can clog the blood vessels that nourish the brain. Trans fats deliver a double whammy. Not only do they raise artery-clogging blood cholesterol, but trans fats can worm their way into cell membranes where they wreak havoc with the membrane's ability to remain pliable and flexible. In short, trans fats lead to more rigid cell membranes. This limits the ability of brain cells to take up valuable nutrients, expel metabolic byproducts and perform at their best.

Saturated fats

The main sources of saturated fats are foods from animals and a few plants. For example, beef, beef fat, veal, lamb, pork, lard, chicken fat, butter, cream, milk, cheese and other dairy products contain saturated fats. Plant foods high in saturated fats include tropical oils like coconut and palm oil.

Trans fats

The second type of fat that can clog arteries and harm brain cells are trans fats. As you just learned, trans fats not only increase the risk for heart disease and other diseases, but are also taken up by brain cells, distort cell membranes and disrupt their ability to communicate.[4]

Trans fats make their way into foods in one of two ways. First, a small amount naturally occurs in some meat and dairy products like beef, lamb, butter and cheese. This naturally occurring form doesn't have the adverse health effects that industrially produced trans fats do. In fact, naturally occurring trans fats may even have a protective effect.[5]

The real culprit is artificially produced trans fats like the partially hydrogenated oils that have been so commonplace in processed foods. Here, a manufacturing process called hydrogenation is used to make a liquid vegetable oil stay semi-solid at room temperature. As you'll learn shortly, partially hydrogenated oil is no longer an approved food ingredient in the U.S.[6] If you think that's a big win for kids' health, you'd be right.

To see how saturated fats and trans fats are listed in the Nutrition Facts panel, check out the example on the next page for a typical milk chocolate creamy frosting.

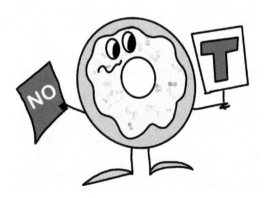

Milk Chocolate Creamy Frosting

Here's where to look for saturated and trans fats.

For some foods, these fats may be listed in the footnote as "Not a significant source," which means less than 0.5 grams per serving.

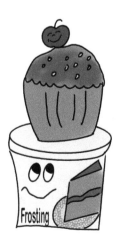

Nutrition Facts

About 13 servings per container

Serving size   **2 tbsp (33g)**

Amount per serving

Calories   130

% Daily Value*

Total Fat 5g	7%
Saturated Fat 2.5g	13%
Trans Fat 0g	
Cholesterol 0mg	0%
Sodium 80mg	4%
Total Carbohydrate 21g	8%
Dietary Fiber 0g	0%
Total Sugars 17g	
Includes 17g Added Sugars	33%
Protein 0g	
Iron 0.5mg	2%

Not a significant source of vitamin D, calcium and potassium.

* The % Daily Value tells you how much a nutrient in a serving of food contributes to a daily diet. 2,000 calories a day is used for general nutrition advice.

Ingredients: Sugar, Water, **Palm Oil**, Corn Syrup, Corn Starch, Cocoa Processed with Alkali. Contains 2% or Less of: Salt, Monoglycerides, Polysorbate 60, Sodium Stearoyl Lactylate, Sodium Acid Pyrophosphate, Citric Acid, Natural and Artificial Flavor. Freshness Preserved by Potassium Sorbate.

Terrible with a capital "T"

Trans fats are more harmful to your health than saturated fats, so much so that health experts recommend you keep your intake as low as possible and not exceed 1% of your daily calories since higher levels adversely affect heart health.[7] In practical terms, this means no more than 1 to 3 grams of trans fats per day for kids (and adults), depending on calorie needs. In other words, there's no place in a healthy diet for industrially produced artificial trans fats.

FDA bans partially hydrogenated oil

There's no doubt about it, partially hydrogenated oil can improve food texture and flavor and even help extend shelf life, plus it's cheap. So, it's easy to see why it has been used in so many processed foods. Think cookies, pies and other baked goods, margarines, fried potatoes, fried chicken, microwave popcorn, fast foods and restaurant foods.[8] In fact, the vast majority of trans fats in the diet comes from the partially hydrogenated oil found in these and other processed foods. That is, until June 2018, when the FDA revoked its "Generally Recognized as Safe" (GRAS) status.

This regulatory move effectively bans the use of partially hydrogenated oil as a food ingredient. With three years to comply, the food industry has been slowly removing this culprit from the food supply and replacing it with less harmful fats like palm oil, palm kernel oil, coconut oil and other oils.[9]

Larger manufacturers had until January 1, 2020 to comply, smaller ones were given an extra year, and some single-ingredient foods had until July 1, 2021 to do so. Accounting for shelf life, this means most foods on grocery shelves should now be free of partially hydrogenated oil and labeled with the updated Nutrition Facts panel.

A word of caution

While the replacement oils are free of trans fats, some may be higher in saturated fat. For this reason, you'll need to keep your labeling reading skills sharp and scan the Nutrition Facts panel to see whether the amount of saturated fats went up as the amount of trans fats went down.

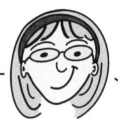

Did You Know?

Since the U.S. Food and Drug Administration's 2018 ban on partially hydrogenated oils in foods, manufacturers are turning to palm oil. This oil is semi-solid at room temperature, so it works well as a substitute for partially hydrogenated oil in many products. Plus, it's cheap. Trouble is, to meet the increase in demand, palm oil plantations are expanding, particularly in high-producing countries like Indonesia and Malaysia. In the process, they're destroying rainforest habitats that are home to endangered species. For this reason, environmental advocates urge food companies to minimize the use of palm oil or, at the very least, use sustainable sources.[10]

Guideline 6: Choose Low-Sodium Foods More Often

Kids who eat a typical American diet tend to consume too much sodium, which can send blood pressure racing skyward and increase the risk of heart disease and kidney disease. Since processed and packaged foods top the list of high-sodium foods in the American diet, your label reading skills could make a big dent in your child's sodium intake. And, remember that healthy habits described in other chapters like eating more fruits and veggies, maintaining a healthy body weight and staying active also help keep blood pressure in the healthy range.

Just how much sodium is considered healthy?

Younger kids, age 4 to 8 years, need to limit sodium intake to no more than 1,500 milligrams per day, while older kids, 9 to 13 years, need to limit their intake to no more than 1,800 milligrams per day, according to the 2020-2025 Dietary Guidelines for Americans.[3] In practical terms, that's less than a teaspoon of salt. Compare that to the typical sodium intake, which is much higher for both younger kids (about 2,500 milligrams per day) and older kids (about 2,900 milligrams per day).[11]

Look beyond the salt shaker

Sodium isn't just in table salt (sodium chloride). In fact, the salt shaker is a minor contributor to total sodium intake compared to the sodium found in just about every category of food as monosodium glutamate (MSG), sodium bicarbonate, sodium nitrite or other forms. The good news is you need only look at the Nutrition Facts panel to find the amount of sodium per serving regardless of its source. Checking the Nutrition Facts panel is an especially good way to compare the sodium content of similar packaged foods like soups that can vary by several hundred milligrams for the same serving size.

Another option is to look for packaged foods with front-of-package claims such as "low sodium" or "very low sodium." The FDA restricts the use of the term "low sodium" to packaged foods with no more than 140 milligrams of sodium per serving (6% of the Daily Value). The term "very low sodium" has stricter guidelines and is limited to packaged foods with no more than 35 milligrams of sodium per serving (less than 2% of the Daily Value).

As a rule, always double check the Nutrition Facts panel for a food with front-of-package claims such as "salt-free," "unsalted," or "without added salt." While the FDA regulates these terms as well, they only mean no salt is added during processing. The sodium content of the food may still be high due to naturally occurring sodium or sodium-containing additives.

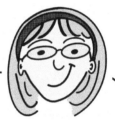

Did You Know?

You can lower your sodium intake dramatically by draining and rinsing canned beans and vegetables with water. In one analysis, America's Test Kitchen sent cans of chickpeas, cannellini beans, pinto beans and black beans to a food lab to find out just how much sodium gets washed away. Turns out, this simple step is well worth the effort. In each case, draining and rinsing the beans reduced sodium by up to 27% (about 100 milligrams per one-half cup serving). Learn more at www.americastestkitchen.com.

Regular vs. Low-Sodium Tomato Soup

Nutrition Facts

1 serving per container

Serving size   **1 Container**
(7.25 oz. low sodium)

Amount per serving

Calories   90

	% Daily Value*
Total Fat 1g	1%
Saturated Fat 0.5g	3%
Trans Fat 0g	
Polyunsaturated Fat 0.5g	
Monounsaturated Fat 0.5g	
Cholesterol less than 5mg	2%
Sodium 790mg	34%
Total Carbohydrate 18g	7%
Dietary Fiber 1g	4%
Total Sugars 10g	
Includes 6g Added Sugars	12%
Protein 2g	
Vitamin D 0mcg	0%
Calcium 20mg	0%
Iron 0.5mg	2%
Potassium 230mg	4%

* The % Daily Value tells you how much a nutrient in a serving of food contributes to a daily diet. 2,000 calories a day is used for general nutrition advice.

> Look here for sodium content.
> Regular (left); low-sodium (right)

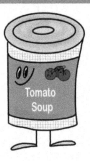

Nutrition Facts

1 serving per container

Serving size   **1 Container**
(7.25 oz. low sodium)

Amount per serving

Calories   110

	% Daily Value*
Total Fat 1g	1%
Saturated Fat 0.5g	3%
Trans Fat 0g	
Polyunsaturated Fat 0.5g	
Monounsaturated Fat 0.5g	
Cholesterol less than 5mg	2%
Sodium 50mg	2%
Total Carbohydrate 22g	8%
Dietary Fiber 2g	0%
Total Sugars 15g	
Includes 10g Added Sugars	20%
Protein 0g	
Vitamin D 0mcg	0%
Calcium 20mg	0%
Iron 0.9mg	4%
Potassium 50mg	6%

* The % Daily Value tells you how much a nutrient in a serving of food contributes to a daily diet. 2,000 calories a day is used for general nutrition advice.

Using your sodium know-how

You can test your label reading skills on two kid-friendly foods that are notorious for being high in sodium: soup and hard pretzels. During your next trip to the grocery store, take a look at both regular and low-sodium varieties. You just may be surprised at the dramatic difference in sodium content. For example, compare the Nutrition Facts panels for a typical regular and a low-sodium tomato soup on the previous page, and you'll quickly see the difference. The regular, ready-to-serve tomato soup has almost 800 milligrams of sodium (34% of the Daily Value) per one-cup serving. Switch to the low-sodium variety, and you cut the sodium to 50 milligrams per one-cup serving (2% of the Daily Value).

Note: Sugar is often added to offset the loss in flavor that occurs when you remove salt, so check for added sugars as well. Apply the same strategy to choosing a brand of hard pretzels, and you can cut the sodium content from over 300 milligrams per one-ounce serving of the salted variety to zero for some unsalted versions. Remember, each lower sodium choice moves you one step closer to controlling your child's sodium intake, so start applying your label reading skills today.

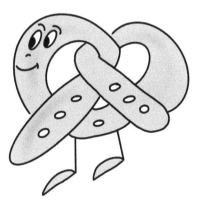

Cinnamon Oats Granola

Look here for the amounts of total and added sugars.

The Ingredient list is where the common names for any sources of sugar are listed.

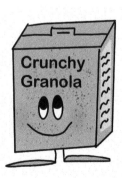

Nutrition Facts

About 5 servings per container

Serving size	**2/3 cup (65g)**

Amount per serving

Calories   240

	% Daily Value*
Total Fat 7g	**9%**
Saturated Fat 0.5g	**3%**
Trans Fat 0g	
Polyunsaturated Fat 2.5g	
Monounsaturated Fat 3g	
Cholesterol 0mg	**0%**
Sodium 50mg	**2%**
Total Carbohydrate 42g	**15%**
Dietary Fiber 9g	**32%**
Total Sugars 10g	
Includes 9g Added Sugars	**18%**
Protein 5g	
Vitamin D 0mcg	0%
Calcium 37mg	2%
Iron 2mg	10%
Potassium 184mg	4%

* The % Daily Value tells you how much a nutrient in a serving of food contributes to a daily diet. 2,000 calories a day is used for general nutrition advice.

Ingredients: Oats, **Cane Sugar**, Brown Rice, Chicory Root Fiber, Flax Seed, Canola Oil, Buckwheat, Millet, Amaranth, **Molasses**, Cinnamon, Quinoa, **Brown Rice Syrup**, Sea Salt, Vitamin E (Tocopherols to Maintain Freshness).

Guideline 7: Know the Sweet Lingo

Sugars naturally occur in fruits, grains, milk and milk products, but sugars are also added to packaged foods for a variety of reasons. They impart a sweet taste, but in many foods, added sugars also help improve texture and appearance. Trouble is, consuming too much can sap your child's brain power and increase their risk for obesity, type 2 diabetes, kidney diseases and other metabolic diseases. Plus, added sugars are notorious for eroding tooth enamel and increasing tooth decay.[12] That's a big price to pay for a little sweetness.

An easier way to say goodbye to added sugars

Along with other changes, the updated Nutrition Facts panel now includes a separate entry for the amount of added sugars in a packaged food. And, the listing is mandatory. That's good news if you want an easier way to see whether the sugar is naturally present in a food or added.

Of course, food manufactures are still required to list the sources of added sugars in a packaged food in the Ingredient list. (Remember, this is the statement right below the Nutrition Facts panel.) Like the Nutrition Facts panel, the Ingredient list is highly regulated so no marketing tomfoolery allowed here. Rather, it's an ordinary list of ingredients using common or usual names. You can continue to use this with confidence to find the sources of added sugars. Be sure to notice where they are positioned in the Ingredient list. It's important because the FDA requires manufacturers to list ingredients in descending order by weight. So, if sugar (or another term for added sugars) is listed among the first three ingredients, the food is likely high in added sugars.

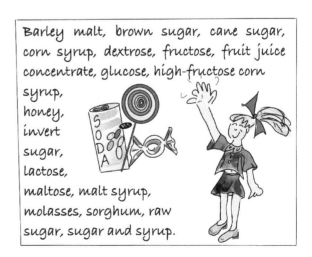

Barley malt, brown sugar, cane sugar, corn syrup, dextrose, fructose, fruit juice concentrate, glucose, high-fructose corn syrup, honey, invert sugar, lactose, maltose, malt syrup, molasses, sorghum, raw sugar, sugar and syrup.

Since granola is notorious for added sugars, let's look at an example. On page 220, you'll find the Nutrition Facts panel and Ingredient list for a typical granola cereal. With the updated Nutrition Facts panel, you can see one 2/3 cup serving contains 10 grams of total sugars of which 90% (9 grams) are added sugars. When you look at the Ingredient list, you can see why. It contains cane sugar (the second ingredient by weight), molasses and brown rice syrup.

A word about sugar alcohols

Mannitol, sorbitol, xylitol and other sugar alcohols are also popular sweeteners. These ingredients are produced commercially from various sugars. Sugar alcohols are absorbed from the digestive tract more slowly than sugar, which makes them a good choice for special dietary foods. They also tend to be less likely to cause tooth decay. However, when consumed in large amounts, sugar alcohols can have a laxative effect and cause digestive upset in sensitive people, which limits their use in foods.

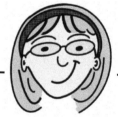

Did You Know?

Chewing gums that contain sugar alcohols help reduce plaque and mouth bacteria. This could mean fewer cavities and a brighter smile. Look for the "ol" at the end of the ingredient names. These include xylit<u>ol</u>, sorbit<u>ol</u> and mannit<u>ol</u>. Of the three, xylitol has the greatest promise for cavity prevention.

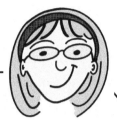

Did You Know?

There are many terms for added sugar in packaged foods. Luckily, common and usual names are required to be used in a food label's Ingredient statement, making them easier to recognize. Here are a few:

Brown sugar	Invert sugar
Corn sweetener	Lactose
Corn syrup	Maltose
Dextrose	Malt syrup
Fructose	Molasses
Fruit juice concentrate	Raw sugar
Glucose	Sucrose
High-fructose corn syrup	Sugar
Honey	Syrup

Black Bean Vegetarian Chili

Look here for dietary fiber. Foods with at least 6 grams (20% of the Daily Value) or more per serving are high in fiber, like this hearty vegetarian chili.

Nutrition Facts

2 servings per container

Serving size   **1 cup (245g)**

Amount per serving

Calories   210

% Daily Value*

Total Fat 2.5g	**3%**
Saturated Fat 0g	**0%**
Trans Fat 0g	
Cholesterol 0mg	**0%**
Sodium 650mg	**28%**
Total Carbohydrate 38g	**14%**
Dietary Fiber 9g	**32%**
Total Sugars 7g	
Protein 9g	
Calcium 90mg	6%
Iron 3.4mg	20%
Potassium 780mg	15%

Not a significant source of trans fat, cholesterol, added sugars and vitamin D.

* The % Daily Value tells you how much a nutrient in a serving of food contributes to a daily diet. 2,000 calories a day is used for general nutrition advice.

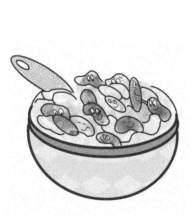

Guideline 8: Focus on High-Fiber Foods

Children need high-fiber foods to keep their digestion and elimination in tip-top shape—which means fewer visits to the pediatrician. High-fiber foods not only help promote digestive and heart health, but also help maintain steady blood sugar levels. What's more, this versatile nutrient offers a bonus for overweight kids. How? High-fiber foods are filling, so kids eat less, but still feel satisfied.

You'll find fiber in plant-based foods such as fruits, vegetables, dried beans and peas, nuts and whole grains. This wide variety of choices makes it even easier to include at least one high-fiber food at every meal.

How much is enough?

Just how much fiber do children need? As a rule of thumb, kids (and adults) should consume 14 grams of fiber for every 1,000 calories they eat. Younger kids, 4 to 8 years old, should aim for about 25 grams per day, while older kids, 9 to 13 years old, should aim for about 26 to 31 grams of fiber daily.

Look for "6" for high-fiber foods

When it comes to packaged foods, you can quickly find the fiber content. If a food contains enough fiber worth mentioning, you'll find it prominently listed in the Nutrition Facts panel. And, if the food contains at least 5.6 grams of fiber per serving, it's earned the right to be called a "high-fiber" food because that's at least 20% of the Daily Value. (On product labels, this rounds up to 6 grams of fiber per serving.) In this case, you're likely to also see a big, bold banner across the front of the package extolling the high-fiber virtues of the product.

Guideline 9: Not All Organic Products Are Alike

If you're interested in choosing organic foods for your family, then you'll want to keep an eye out for packaged foods with the USDA Organic Seal. The U.S. Department of Agriculture (USDA) allows manufacturers to use this seal on packaging when foods are made with 100% organic ingredients. However, the USDA also allows three other types of organic label claims for foods that have some—but not all—organic ingredients.

The four levels of "organic"

Here's the breakdown of the USDA's organic claims permitted for use on foods:

- **100% Organic.** Just as the claim suggests, these foods are completely organic and qualify to use the USDA Organic Seal.
- **Organic.** The contents of foods with this claim must be at least 95% organic by weight, excluding water and salt. These foods also qualify to use the USDA Organic Seal.
- **Made With Organic.** At least 70% of the contents of foods with this claim must be organic. You'll likely find the "Made with Organic" claim splashed across the front of the package, but the USDA Organic Seal is not permitted on these foods.
- **Less than 70% of content is organic.** Foods that meet this criterion may only list ingredients that are organic in the Ingredient panel. These foods are not permitted to mention organic on the main panel and may not display the USDA Organic Seal.

Organic animal foods

Meats, eggs and dairy products may be labeled organic when producers follow a few key rules. First, they must allow the animals outside. Second, they cannot give animals growth hormones or antibiotics. Finally, producers must use animal feed that's organic and free of any parts of other slaughtered animals.

This Month's Smart Goal

I will help my child find high-fiber foods by looking for at least 6 grams of fiber per serving in the Nutrition Facts panel.

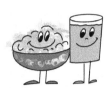

This Month's Extra Credit

While grocery shopping, I will make a game out of seeing how many products my child can find with the USDA Organic Seal for a fun way to learn about organic foods.

To monitor your daily progress toward your goals, use the **My Smart Tracker** forms in **Chapter 14: Go for the Goal.**

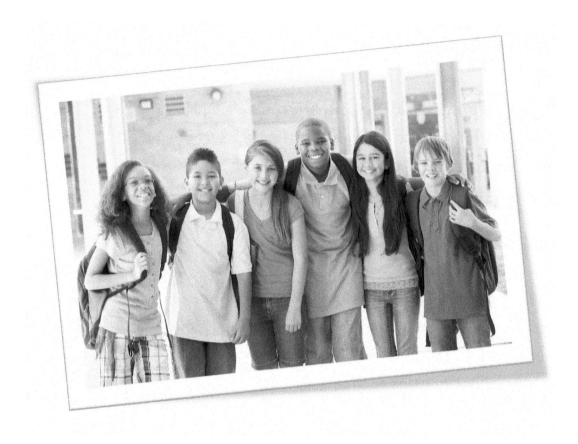

Good habits, once established,
are just as hard to break as are bad habits.
— Robert Puller

Chapter 13

August – Prep for a New School Year

For most parents of young children, August means back-to-school shopping. Whether your child's school clothes are standard issue uniforms or outfits that allow for more self-expression, a quick inventory of last year's wardrobe is sure to confirm the inevitable: Your child has outgrown, well, just about everything.

It's a growth spurt that's easy to spot. You may have noticed your child's face has matured along with a tighter jaw line and a smile that now sports more permanent teeth. It's an incredible transformation.

Even more incredible is the physical change occurring in your child's brain as the complex circuitry of dendrites, axons and other brain cells work to activate learning and memory. You can help ensure that your child's brain stays fueled and ready to learn throughout the new school year by adding a few simple items to your back-to-school shopping list and school routine.

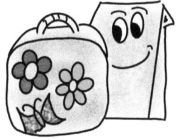

Lunch Box Essentials

Packing a lunch becomes much easier when you have the proper supplies on hand. So, when shopping for school supplies, don't forget to add the following lunch essentials:

1 **Lunch box.** Young kids love getting a new lunch box with the latest cartoon character, action figure or other popular design. Whatever the choice, make sure it's both sturdy and easy to clean. Also, remember to write your child's name in it using a permanent marker in case it gets lost on the playground.

2 **Cold packs.** Cold packs are a must. It only takes a few hours for a non-refrigerated lunch to start growing harmful bacteria that can cause food-borne illnesses and make your child sick. What's more, chilled foods allowed to sit at room temperature tend to go straight to the trash. Warm string cheese, anyone? Consider purchasing several cold packs so you always have one in the freezer ready for use. Some even come in fun shapes such as soccer balls, baseballs and flowers.

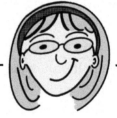

Did You Know?

The U.S. Department of Agriculture (USDA) provides an interactive online tool called "MyPlate." With a click of the mouse, you can get a personalized meal plan that's right for your child. This free tool is available at www.myplate.gov and is based on the 2020-2025 Dietary Guidelines for Americans.[1]

3 **Thermos.** Be sure to purchase two high-quality thermoses, one for beverages and another for food. The best choices are those made from stainless steel. For food, choose a small one (about 10 ounces) with a wide mouth so your child can see what's inside. Make sure it can safely store hot foods for up to 6 hours.

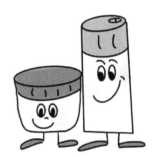

4 **Containers for sandwiches and snacks.** Sturdy containers for sandwiches and other snacks are a plus. You'll avoid overusing disposable baggies, which is friendly to both your budget and the environment.

5 **Stickers, jokes or fancy napkins.** Don't forget to pack a little fun in your child's lunch box. Keep a stash of jokes, riddles and bright stickers on hand for plenty of options to lighten the noontime meal. Be sure to mix it up to keep your child guessing. That's half the fun. It's a no-fuss way to keep your child smiling throughout the new school year.

Easing into the School Year

With the start of school only a few weeks away, consider some of the following tips to make sure your youngster gets off on the right foot.

Get organized

Place all upcoming events like ice cream socials, back-to-school nights, PTA meetings, sports events, scout functions and other activities on a central calendar. Organize a homework niche for your child, and double up on school supplies so that you can keep one set here.

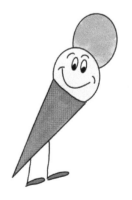

Sweet slumber

If your child has been enjoying a more relaxed bedtime schedule during the summer months, it's time to ease back into a structured routine in preparation for school. After all, optimal learning demands an alert mind that only a good night's sleep can provide. About two weeks before the start of school, start adjusting your child's bedtime hour to mesh with the upcoming school year. Typically, most preschoolers should sleep 10 to 13 hours per day, while children 6 to 12 years of age need at least 9 hours of sleep per day. That means, if your fifth grader wakes up at 6:30 a.m. during school days, aim for a bedtime—and lights out—no later than 9:00 p.m. to allow 30 minutes for sleep to set in.[2]

The "night before" habit

The more you can do the night before a school day, the less chaotic the morning will be. Teach your child to place everything he or she needs for the next school day by the front door. This includes homework neatly tucked inside their backpack. Also, encourage your child to layout the next day's outfit.

The afternoon snack

After long school days, your child is likely to arrive home with a rumbling stomach. An after-school snack is a great routine to help your child replenish his or her energy level after a full day of mental and physical activity. With a little planning, you can be prepared to offer healthy snacks. Fresh cut fruit, a quesadilla made with a whole wheat tortilla or a whole grain bagel with peanut butter are a few snack ideas that can help curb hunger and refuel your child to tackle the day's homework.

Backpack Know-How

An online search for "backpack safety" will send you on your way to a whole host of credible online websites filled with expert tips from the American Academy of Pediatrics to the National Safety Council to the American Physical Therapy Association.

What's more, the American Occupational Therapy Association celebrates their annual National School Backpack Awareness Day on the third Wednesday in September when these ergonomic experts offer safety tips for students, parents, educators, school administrators and community members alike.

While experts continue to debate the finer points of backpack safety, all of them agree on three critical actions you can take to protect your child's health. First, you'll want to choose the right backpack for your child's size. Next, you'll want to teach your child how to pack it for back comfort. Finally, you'll want to encourage your child to wear it properly. In other words, the right size, packed and worn the right way. Focus on these basics and your child is sure to enjoy better back comfort throughout the day and have fewer aches and pains that can distract from learning.

Five Basics for Choosing a Backpack

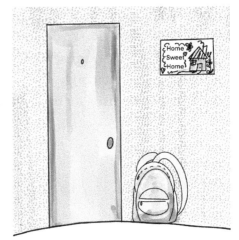

1 Look for sturdy, lightweight construction. The school year can be tough on your child's backpack. After all, it not only needs to survive the daily toting of textbooks and other school supplies, but also the drop-and-toss style of most energetic kids. With the typical school year lasting about 180 days, all those snaps, clasps, zippers and seams take a beating, which is why choosing a sturdy, well-constructed backpack is essential. A sturdy backpack that's also lighter in weight is best, as you want the backpack itself to contribute as little weight as possible.

2 **Consider a trendy design.** While you're looking for a backpack that's sturdy and well-constructed, your child has an eye on one with a trendy color or design. Blend the best of both worlds by encouraging your child to be part of the decision. With so much variety in the market, you can easily select a sturdy brand that's perfectly sized for your child's height and weight in a color or design that they prefer. The result: A sturdy backpack that your child will want to wear.

3 **Make sure shoulder straps are comfortable.** Backpacks with two straps that are wide and padded allow your child to carry their pack across both shoulders. This helps evenly distribute the weight, making it more comfortable. By contrast, carrying a backpack over one shoulder can lead to fatigue, poor posture and lower back pain that can stifle learning. When adjusting the straps, make sure the backpack rests on the curve of your child's back. It should sit 1 to 2 inches below shoulder level on the curve of the back and never more than 4 inches below the belly button.

4 **Choose a padded back.** A padded back certainly offers your child more comfort, but it also protects the body from pencils, pens and other sharp objects that can accidentally puncture through and cause harm.

5 **Pack smart to ease back strain.** Experts tend to agree on how to organize the contents of the backpack: Place the heaviest items on the bottom, in the center and closest to the back. The debate continues, however, on how much weight your child should carry. As a general rule, children should carry backpacks that weigh no more than 15% of their body weight. Keep the load light by encouraging your child to pack only items used for the day.

Backpack Weight Check

Fill your child's backpack for a typical school day and weigh it on a bathroom scale. Weigh your child separately. Compare your child's backpack with the recommended weight limit listed below. Is it time to lighten the load?

Your Child's Body Weight	Backpack Weight Limit (no more than)
50 lbs	7.5 lbs
55 lbs	8.25 lbs
60 lbs	9.0 lbs
65 lbs	9.75 lbs
70 lbs	10.5 lbs
75 lbs	11.25 lbs
80 lbs	12.0 lbs
85 lbs	12.75 lbs
90 lbs	13.5 lbs
95 lbs	14.25 lbs
100 lbs	15 lbs

Source: Backpack safety. American Academy of Pediatrics. https://healthychildren.org.

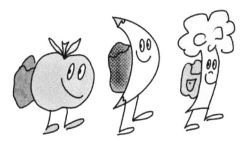

Better Homework

With the official kickoff of the typical school year just a few short weeks away, August is the perfect time to prepare for the daily ritual of homework. Why? Establishing a regular routine—with the emphasis on regular—is essential for developing good study habits that are sure to help your child enjoy learning and breeze through their assignments.

What's more, getting "homework ready" is a lot easier than you may think thanks to the experts at the American Academy of Pediatrics who have compiled a checklist to help you establish a daily homework routine.[3] Read on for a summary of some of these need-to-know basics—along with our practical tips—that are sure to help maximize your child's learning throughout the year.

1 **Establish a space for homework.** A workspace in the home that offers privacy is ideal whether it's your child's bedroom, a quiet corner of the kitchen or other part of the home. A dedicated space is ideal; but, when it's not an option, consider establishing a quiet time for the entire house, a sort of "virtual space" free of distractions that can disrupt homework time.

2 **Set aside plenty of time for homework.** Nothing saps effective learning like stress. By scheduling enough time to complete homework assignments without undue stress, you'll create a relaxed, calm environment that's likely to promote better learning.

3 **Establish a "house rule" to turn the TV off during homework time.** This is especially true when your child's homework space is within earshot of a noisy and distracting TV program. The bonus is scheduled quiet time for you.

4 **Consider a tutor for tough subjects.** If your child is having a challenge with a particular subject, consider enlisting the services of a tutor. A tutor may offer a fresh approach to learning that can help your child more easily understand a difficult subject. Discuss this option with your child's teacher who is likely to be a great resource for suggestions.

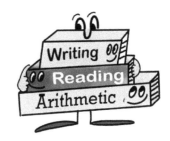

5 **Encourage your child to take regular breaks.** Regular breaks are especially important to prevent eye fatigue and neck strain. Closing the books for a few minutes and stretching also goes a long way to maintain focus and interest.

6 **Be available to answer questions and offer assistance, but avoid doing your child's homework.** This homework must-do is often easier said than done. After all, explaining a new math concept or grammar rule typically takes a bit more patience and time, but your extra effort will pay off with a child who is not only more proficient in a particular subject, but also likely to be more confident and self-assured.

7 **Supervise computer and Internet use.** When used properly, the Internet is a great educational tool for kids. It offers ready access to numerous resources for school projects from digital textbooks and other materials posted by teachers to interactive team projects with classmates. Trouble is, it's just as easy to navigate to the latest online game or to other distractions. By keeping a watchful eye on computer time, you can help your child stay focused on what matters: homework.

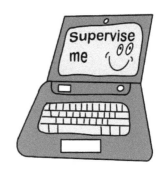

This Month's Smart Goal

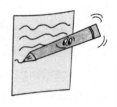

At least two weeks before school starts,
I will establish a homework space based
on the "Better Homework" tips.

This Month's Extra Credit

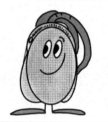

At least two weeks before school starts,
I will buy a backpack based on the
"Backpack Know-How" tips.

To monitor your daily progress toward your goals, use the **My Smart Tracker** forms in **Chapter 14: Go for the Goal.**

Part 6

Extras

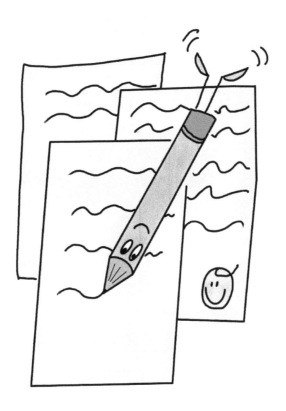

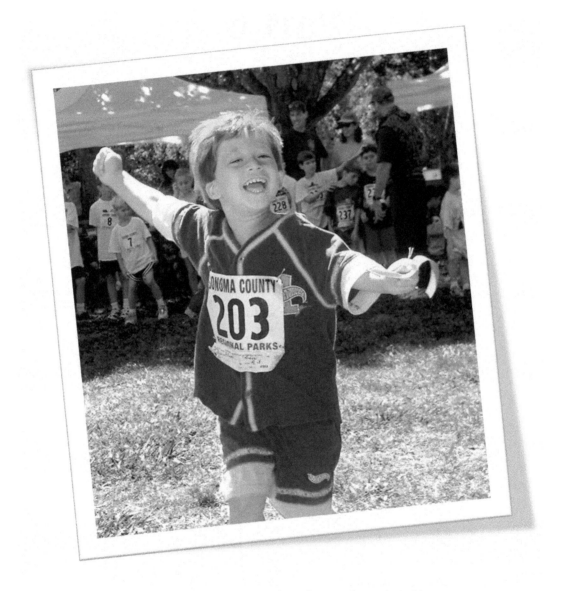

A goal properly set is halfway reached.
– Abraham Lincoln

Chapter 14

Go for the Goal

One of the most effective ways to keep your daily motivation up as you work toward shaping the healthy habits your child needs to be smarter and healthier is to track progress. That's what this chapter is all about: fast and easy goal tracking.

Here you'll find **My Smart Tracker** forms. These pre-printed monthly tracking forms correspond to each chapter's goal and extra credit. We've also included plenty of blank forms to inspire you to track even more healthy habits.

Ready to get started? Here's how: Turn to the monthly goal you want to work on. Fill in the corresponding dates for the month. Now you're ready to track. At the end of the day, you simply grab a pen and check off whether you've made progress toward the goal.

Don't underestimate the power of this simple, yet elegant tool. Few things are more motivating than seeing regular progress, especially for health-related goals.

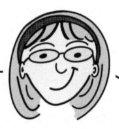

Did You Know?

Tracking your daily progress toward your SMART goals is the first step to your success. But don't forget to reflect on your monthly success. At the end of each month, write down a short sentence or two about the progress you've made toward your monthly goal and any thoughts you may have about your success. Seeing your progress in writing is a great confidence booster that helps keep motivation high and goals on track.

September | Goal

I will add one family meal each week to reach
at least five per week.*

*At least five is the goal, but for this goal and all others, start where
you and your family are. A goal shouldn't be too hard (or too easy).

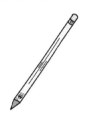

SUN	MON	TUE	WED	THU	FRI	SAT

This month I accomplished: _____
_____
_____

Notes: _____
_____
_____
_____

September | Extra Credit

I will give my child a children's multivitamin with iron every day, preferably at breakfast.

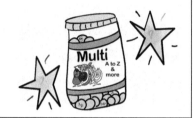

SUN	MON	TUE	WED	THU	FRI	SAT

This month I accomplished: _____

_____

_____

Notes: _____

_____

_____

_____

October | Goal

I will serve breakfast every day and include a protein-rich food.

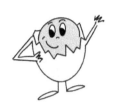

SUN	MON	TUE	WED	THU	FRI	SAT

This month I accomplished: _____

_____

_____

Notes: _____

_____

_____

_____

October | Extra Credit

I will give my child a DHA supplement every day, preferably at breakfast.

SUN	MON	TUE	WED	THU	FRI	SAT

This month I accomplished: _____

_____

_____

Notes: _____

_____

_____

_____

November | Goal

I will add one serving of fruits or vegetables each week until my child meets the recommended intake (at least 3 to 5 servings daily based on age).

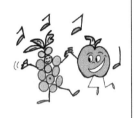

SUN	MON	TUE	WED	THU	FRI	SAT

This month I accomplished: _____

_____

_____

Notes: _____

_____

_____

_____

November | Extra Credit

I will serve a fruit or veggie in each color group (purple, red, orange-yellow, green and white-brown) every day.*

*While every day is preferable, start with where you are and slowly build up.

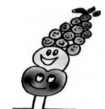

SUN	MON	TUE	WED	THU	FRI	SAT

This month I accomplished: _____

_____

_____

Notes: _____

_____

_____

_____

December | Goal

I will enforce a regular bedtime hour to help my child get enough memory-enhancing REM sleep at least five times per week.

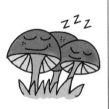

SUN	MON	TUE	WED	THU	FRI	SAT

This month I accomplished: _____

_____

_____

Notes: _____

_____

_____

_____

December | Extra Credit

I will have my child take at least 5 minutes a day to stop, listen and learn (and really "bee" present in the moment).

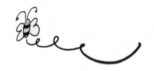

SUN	MON	TUE	WED	THU	FRI	SAT

This month I accomplished: _____

_____

_____

Notes: _____

_____

_____

_____

January | Goal

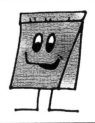

I will have my child help with the planning and making of school lunches at least once a week.

SUN	MON	TUE	WED	THU	FRI	SAT

This month I accomplished: _____
_____
_____

Notes: _____
_____
_____
_____

January | Extra Credit

I will include a joke, riddle, brainteaser or other fun pick in my child's lunch box at least twice a week.

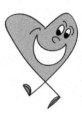

SUN	MON	TUE	WED	THU	FRI	SAT

This month I accomplished: _____

_____

_____

Notes: _____

_____

_____

_____

February | Goal

I will have my child help create one complete meal for the family this month (grocery shopping, cooking and setting the table).

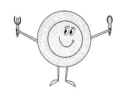

SUN	MON	TUE	WED	THU	FRI	SAT

This month I accomplished: _____
_____
_____

Notes: _____
_____
_____
_____

February | Extra Credit

I will play Rate Your Plate with my child at three meals per week (and earn at least 5 points per session).

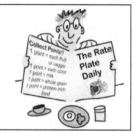

SUN	MON	TUE	WED	THU	FRI	SAT

This month I accomplished: _____

_____

_____

Notes: _____

_____

_____

_____

March | Goal

I will add 5 minutes of jumping, running or other fun activity until my child is active at least 60 minutes every day. (Take it one step at a time, listen to your child, and make sure it's fun.)

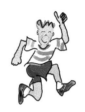

SUN	MON	TUE	WED	THU	FRI	SAT

This month I accomplished: _____

_____

_____

Notes: _____

_____

_____

_____

March | Extra Credit

I will help my child play outside in full sunlight at least 2 hours each day to promote healthy vision.

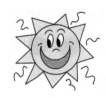

SUN	MON	TUE	WED	THU	FRI	SAT

This month I accomplished: _____

_____

_____

Notes: _____

_____

_____

_____

April | Goal

I will help my child brainstorm a healthier substitute for one of their frequent junk food choices this month.

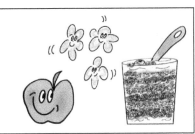

SUN	MON	TUE	WED	THU	FRI	SAT

This month I accomplished: _____

_____

_____

Notes: _____

_____

_____

_____

April | Extra Credit

I will help my child limit sweets to once daily.

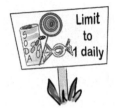

SUN	MON	TUE	WED	THU	FRI	SAT

This month I accomplished: _____

_____

_____

Notes: _____

_____

_____

_____

May | Goal

I will serve at least one new fruit, vegetable or whole grain food each week.

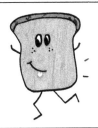

SUN	MON	TUE	WED	THU	FRI	SAT

This month I accomplished: _____

_____

_____

Notes: _____

_____

_____

_____

May | Extra Credit

I will start a "square foot" garden.

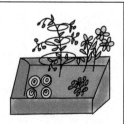

SUN	MON	TUE	WED	THU	FRI	SAT

This month I accomplished: _____

_____

_____

Notes: _____

_____

_____

_____

June | Goal

I will have my child track urine color and drink more water if the color resembles apple juice.

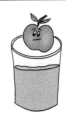

SUN	MON	TUE	WED	THU	FRI	SAT

This month I accomplished: _____
_____
_____

Notes: _____
_____
_____
_____

June | Extra Credit

I will make a summer "To Do" list with my family of activities that stimulate the mind, body and spirit.

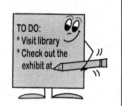

SUN	MON	TUE	WED	THU	FRI	SAT

This month I accomplished: _____

_____

_____

Notes: _____

_____

_____

_____

July | Goal

I will help my child find high-fiber foods by looking for at least 6 grams of fiber per serving in the Nutrition Facts panel.

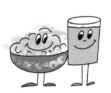

SUN	MON	TUE	WED	THU	FRI	SAT

This month I accomplished: _____
_____
_____

Notes: _____
_____
_____
_____

July | Extra Credit

While grocery shopping, I will make a game out of seeing how many products my child can find with the USDA Organic Seal for a fun way to learn about organic foods.

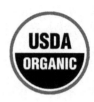

SUN	MON	TUE	WED	THU	FRI	SAT

This month I accomplished: _____

_____

_____

Notes: _____

_____

_____

_____

August | Goal

At least two weeks before school starts,
I will establish a homework space based
on the "Better Homework" tips.

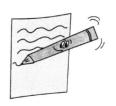

SUN	MON	TUE	WED	THU	FRI	SAT

This month I accomplished: _____
_____
_____

Notes: _____
_____
_____
_____

August | Extra Credit

At least two weeks before school starts, I will buy a backpack based on the "Backpack Know-How" tips.

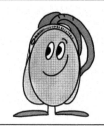

SUN	MON	TUE	WED	THU	FRI	SAT

This month I accomplished: _____
_____
_____

Notes: _____
_____
_____
_____

Month:_____ | Goal

I will _____

_____

_____

SUN	MON	TUE	WED	THU	FRI	SAT

This month I accomplished: _____

_____

_____

Notes: _____

_____

_____

_____

Month:_____ | Goal

I will _____

_____

_____

SUN	MON	TUE	WED	THU	FRI	SAT

This month I accomplished: _____

_____

_____

Notes: _____

_____

_____

_____

Month:_____ | **Goal**

I will _____

_____

_____

SUN	MON	TUE	WED	THU	FRI	SAT

This month I accomplished: _____

_____

_____

Notes: _____

_____

_____

_____

Month:_____ | Goal

I will _____

_____

_____

SUN	MON	TUE	WED	THU	FRI	SAT

This month I accomplished: _____

_____

_____

Notes: _____

_____

_____

_____

Month:_____ | Goal

I will _____

_____

_____

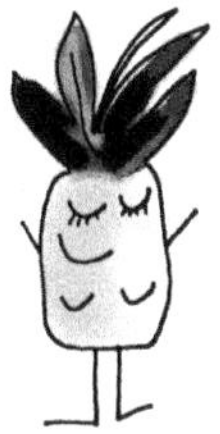

SUN	MON	TUE	WED	THU	FRI	SAT

This month I accomplished: _____

_____

_____

Notes: _____

_____

_____

_____

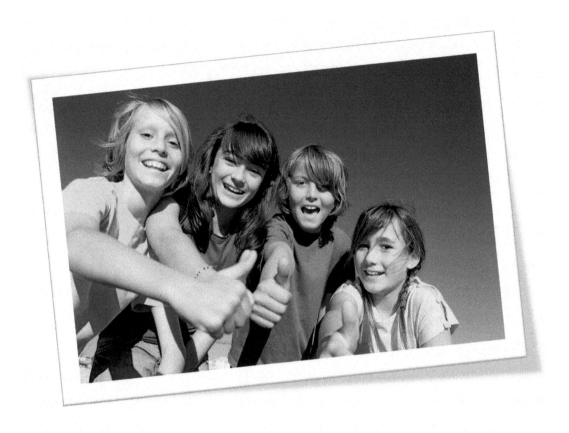

We can all agree that in the wealthiest nation on Earth, all children should have the basic nutrition they need to learn and grow and to pursue their dreams, because in the end, nothing is more important than the health and well-being of our children. Nothing.
— Michelle Obama

Chapter 15

Tables, Tips & More

We know kids don't eat nutrition; they eat enticing foods that taste great. We've got you covered. In this chapter, you'll find with plenty of useful resources to help you fuel your child's growing body and active brain. Here's the list:

- Recipe Makeover Tips & Tricks
- Stocking Your Fridge, Freezer & Pantry
- Choosing Kitchen Utensils & Tools
- Recommended Daily Intake: Calories
- Recommended Daily "Empty Calorie" Limit
- Sample Serving Sizes for Each Food Group
- Recommended Daily Intake: Food Groups
- Recommended Daily Intake: Vitamins
- Recommended Daily Intake: Minerals
- Recommended Daily Intake: Macronutrients
- Recommended Daily Intake: Water

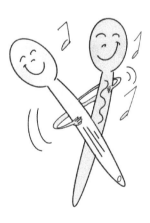

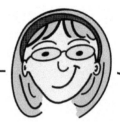

Did You Know?

Compared to conventionally grown crops, organic varieties often have higher antioxidant levels. Organic dairy products are significantly higher in healthy omega-3 fatty acids like EPA and DHA. And, organic meat products have a better nutritional profile. All good reasons to eat more organic foods. But, just as important is what organic foods don't contain. Think a lower load of toxic metabolites, including heavy metals such as cadmium, and synthetic fertilizer and pesticide residues. Plus, eating more organic foods may reduce your child's exposure to antibiotic-resistant bacteria. With so many benefits, it's no surprise researchers report a direct link between better health and replacing conventional foods with organic varieties.[1]

Recipe Makeover Tips & Tricks

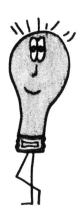

With a few minor adjustments, you can maximize the health benefits of your favorite recipes. The key is to focus on cutting the fat and sugar and boosting the fiber in a way that keeps the flavor impact high. Here are our best kitchen-tested, kid-approved makeover tips to help you pack more nutrition into your favorite recipes. In this way, you can fuel for your child's active brain without compromising flavor.

Tips to Cut Fat

- **Reach for applesauce.** In recipes for most quick breads, muffins or other baked goods, you can replace up to half of the butter, oil or shortening with applesauce or dried plum (prune) puree without dramatically affecting texture.

- **Skip the cream.** Transform creamy sauces into lower fat alternatives by replacing cream with evaporated skim milk, light cream or non-fat half-and-half. Add a little flour as a thickening agent to help maintain a smooth consistency.

- **Use non-toxic, non-stick pans or a cooking oil spray mister.** This simple change will dramatically reduce the amount of fat needed for cooking.

- **Add a rack when roasting.** Placing poultry or meat on a rack will allow the excess fat to drip off.

- **Switch to lower fat dairy products.** Substituting low-fat or non-fat dairy products for whole fat varieties in your recipes will reduce the fat without altering flavor.

- **Cook soups and gravies and refrigerate overnight**. This allows enough time for excess fat to congeal on the top for easy skimming.

- **Substitute with plain yogurt.** Plain yogurt is an ideal substitute for recipes that call for sour cream or mayonnaise.

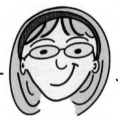

Did You Know?

Dietary fiber is the term that describes material from plant cells the body's enzymes are unable to digest. You won't find fiber in any animal-based foods, not even the toughest steaks. So, when you think of fiber-rich foods, think plant foods. Here's a list of some of the best sources:

- Unrefined, whole grain breads and cereals
- Legumes such as pinto and kidney beans
- Vegetables, especially peas, broccoli, spinach, tomatoes, potatoes, carrots, corn and green peppers
- Fresh fruits with skins or seeds such as apples, apricots, pears, plums and berries

Tips to Cut Sugar

- **Reduce sugar gradually in a recipe.** Most recipes allow for cutting the amount of refined sugar by about one-fourth—and in some cases up to one-third—without affecting taste or texture.

- **Substitute apple juice concentrate for sugar in baked goods.** This is our go-to staple to cut refined sugar in recipes. Here's a good rule-of-thumb: For every one cup of sugar, substitute ¾ cup apple juice concentrate while decreasing the amount of liquid in the recipe by three tablespoons.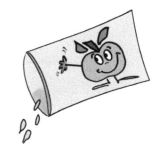

- **Serve sweet foods warm.** Heat enhances the perception of sweetness, helping you to retain the flavor while cutting the sugar.

Tips to Boost Fiber

- **Gradually add more fiber to your child's diet.** This allows the digestive tract to adjust. Adding more dietary fiber too quickly may lead to digestive upset and stomach ache.

- **Choose carbohydrates in their natural fibrous coatings.** For example, brown rice instead of white rice or 100% whole grain crackers, breads and cereals instead of their white counterparts. In many recipes, you can replace up to half of the white flour with a whole grain flour.

- **Serve more vegetables and fruits with edible skins and seeds**. These plant parts are good sources of dietary fiber. Keep a vegetable brush on hand to wash skins during food prep.

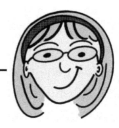

Did You Know?

Frozen fruits and vegetables have an impressive ability to retain their nutritive value. In one study, researchers selected eight common fruits and vegetables including blueberries, broccoli, carrots, corn, green beans, peas, spinach and strawberries. They harvested, processed and analyzed samples at three separate storage times. The nutrients analyzed included vitamins B12, C, E and beta-carotene (a building block for vitamin A). In general, both frozen and fresh varieties had similar amounts of vitamins during the storage period. Beta-carotene, on the other hand, tended to decline more with frozen varieties.[2]

Stocking Your Fridge, Freezer & Pantry

Stocking your kitchen with healthy foods is one of the easiest ways to ensure your child has nutrient-rich choices at the ready when hunger strikes. Read on for a list of staples for your refrigerator, freezer and pantry along with kid-friendly serving suggestions that are sure to please.

Foods for Your Refrigerator

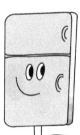

- **Cottage cheese.** Serve with fruit or in salads, or toss with cooked pasta and vegetables with a sprinkle of parmesan cheese.

- **Cheese.** Serve sliced on whole wheat crackers, melted over a whole grain bagel or grated in a fresh salad.

- **Eggs.** Serve poached, scrambled or boiled, and consider buying DHA-enriched eggs for a brain boost.

- **Flax (milled).** Sprinkle on cereal and add in recipes for extra omega-3 protection.

- **Milk.** Pour over cereals, blend into smoothies or enjoy as a nutritious beverage all by itself.

- **Pre-cut veggies and fruit.** Pre-cut and ready to serve makes for a great time saver when hunger strikes.

- **Yogurt (plain or flavored).** Mix with fresh fruit for a yogurt parfait or use a plain variety to replace mayonnaise in salad dressings or sour cream on a baked potato.

Foods for Your Freezer

- **Bread products.** Whole wheat bread and rolls, English muffins and pita bread are kid-friendly and make for fast and healthy options when toasted and topped with cheese, peanut butter, no-added-sugar jams or apple butter.

- **Frozen fruit pieces (with no added sugar).** Use for a quick dessert idea or blend with milk or yogurt for a thick shake.

- **Frozen vegetables (no added cream or butter).** Serve as a side dish, add to pasta or top a baked potato sprinkled with cheese.

- **Frozen fish (such as salmon), chicken or other lean meats.** Stir fry with vegetables, serve on top of a salad or mix with pasta.

- **Frozen ground turkey.** This versatile staple is not only great for a turkey burger, but also for meat loaf, spaghetti sauce and taco filling.

- **Frozen burgers (turkey, veggie or lean meat).** Ideal for a quick meal when you're in a pinch.

- **Frozen fresh herbs (washed).** Toss into a freezer bag, label and date for ready access.

Foods for Your Pantry

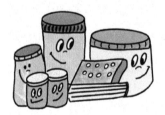

- **Canned tomato products (diced, sauce or paste).** Ideal to add to homemade soups or pasta sauce. Tomato sauce or paste makes an easy topping for a toasted English muffin: simply spread, add grated cheese and broil.

- **Canned tuna, salmon and beans such as pinto, garbanzo and kidney beans.** Drain, rinse and add to salads, soups and stews.

- **Flour.** Keep this recipe staple at the ready; store whole wheat in the refrigerator or freezer to maintain freshness.

- **Grains (whole).** Consider amaranth, brown rice, buckwheat, couscous, kamut, kasha, pasta, quinoa, triticale berries, rye berries, spelt (farro) or wheat berries. Ideal for side dishes, in casseroles or as a topping for stir-fried vegetables.

- **Herbs (assorted) and other flavor enhancers.** Herbs, spices, salt-free seasonings, grated parmesan cheese, vanilla and other extracts are great flavor enhancers to spice up recipes and add variety to your child's diet.

- **Oat bran and oats (rolled or steel-cut).** Serve as breakfast cereal or use in baking.

- **Peanut butter (old-fashioned).** For easier stirring, store the sealed jar upside down until ready to open. This allows the natural oils to move throughout the jar. Refrigerate after opening.

- **Popcorn.** Air-popped as a snack.

- **Potatoes, yams and sweet potatoes.** For an easy, filling meal, bake or microwave and top with vegetables and a protein source. Add to soups and salads or enjoy as leftovers for breakfast. Be sure to store in a cool, dry place.

- **Sugar**. Although you'll likely be using less of this staple in your recipes or sprinkled on foods, it's good to keep some on hand.

- **Unsweetened applesauce, no-sugar-added jams or apple butter.** An ideal substitute for butter as a spread for toast or topping for pancakes.

- **Vegetable oil and vinegar.** For salad dressings and in cooking.

- **Whole wheat crackers.** A quick snack.

Extras

- **Dietary Supplements.** A high-quality children's complete multivitamin/mineral supplement with iron as well as a high-quality omega-3 supplement that provides about 150 to 250 milligrams of EPA + DHA per daily serving.[3] This daily habit helps fill potential nutrient gaps between your child's typical diet and what their active brain needs.

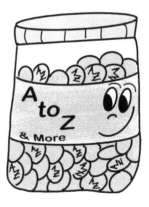

Choosing Kitchen Utensils & Tools

Good tools can make the difference between having fun in the kitchen or sweating away in misery. For this reason, you should aim to buy high-quality items that will last. Read on for a list of need-to-have kitchen utensils and tools (as well as a few nice-to-have choices) and the features that can make your time in the kitchen more enjoyable.

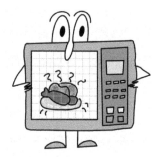

Appliances

- **Blender**. Look for sturdy blades, a rubber base, a glass pitcher and at least one horsepower, especially if smoothies are part of your regular routine.

- **Hand-held beater.** Choose a brand with a case for easy storage of all the parts and pieces that tend to wander.

- **Microwave oven.** Look for an energy-efficient model with a turntable plate, easy-to-read controls, a straight-forward setting sequence and a bright interior light.

- **Pressure Cooker.** Choose a multi-functional electric pressure cooker that has settings for slow cooking, steaming, sauteing, yogurt making and more.

- **Slow Cooker.** Look for a removable pot for easy cleaning, a sturdy base and a timer to prevent overcooking. A 6-quart size is perfect for preparing meals for up to six people.

Bakeware (non-toxic and non-stick)

- **Baking pans.** Most recipes call for an 8- or 9-inch square pan or a 9x12-inch rectangular pan.

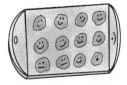

- **Cookie sheets.** Look for low or no sides, a dull finish and a lighter color (to help reduce burning).

- **Loaf pan.** Most recipes for banana, zucchini or other kid-friendly quick breads require a 9x5-inch loaf pan.

- **Muffin tins.** Consider a tin designed for mini muffins for kid-friendly portions.

- **Pie pan.** Consider a pan with an 8- or 9-inch diameter.

Pots and Pans

- **Mixing bowls.** Stainless steel of various sizes that fit within each other for easy storage.

- **Pots.** Stainless steel with covers; most cooks use 1½-quart and 3-quart pots or a 4-quart Dutch oven. For serious homemade soups, consider a 12-quart stock pot.

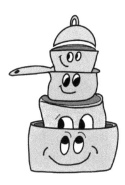

- **Skillets.** Look for stainless steel, iron or non-toxic, non-stick varieties. Consider one small (7-inch diameter) and one large (12-inch diameter) skillet, which would meet most food prep needs.

Gadgets

- **Bottle opener.** Choose a sturdy, old-fashioned style with two ends: one blunt for bottles; the other pointed for cans.

- **Can opener.** Choose a model that cuts around the outside of the can, rather than the lid. The result is a smooth edge and a lid that won't fall into the food.

- **Cheese slicer.** Choose a brand with a sturdy handle. A cheese plane is ideal for hard cheese, while a cheese knife is best for softer varieties.

- **Cookie cutters.** Choose kid-friendly shapes without intricate designs.

- **Cooking thermometer.** Choose an instant, easy-to-read, shatter-proof thermometer with a case.

- **Cutting board.** Wood or plastic (experts have yet to agree on which is more sanitary). Choose the biggest board that your space allows. A smaller one for little jobs may also be helpful.

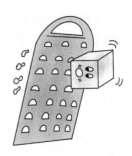

- **Grater.** Best to get at least two: a flat one and a boxed one with different size holes. Plastic graters are safer for children.

- **Ice cube trays.** Choose trays with lids so you can freeze fruit purees for smoothies and vegetable purees for soup stocks.

- **Kitchen knives.** Consider a countertop set that includes a chef's knife, paring knife and a serrated slicing knife.

- **Kitchen shears.** Keep in the kitchen and use only for food items.

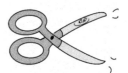

- **Lettuce spinner.** Choose a brand with a plunger rather than a spinner. It's easier on your wrists to spin dry lettuce.

- **Measuring cups.** Choose a brand with a one-piece design and non-collapsible plastic that won't fall apart when full or break if dropped.

- **Measuring spoons.** Choose an oval rather than round shape that's easier to fit into tight spice jars.

- **Peeler.** Choose one that can double as an apple corer.

- **Spatulas.** Consider having a metal one to handle delicate items such as cookies and a rubber one for heavier items such as burgers.

- **Timer.** Choose a digital model with a multiple timekeeping function to track more than one food like a roast in the oven, potatoes on the stove and rising dough on the counter.

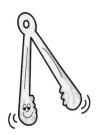

- **Tongs.** Look for fluid movement and not-too-tight spring tension. Examine the tips and make sure they are no more than 6 inches apart to make them less tiresome to hold.

- **Utensils.** Look for dishwasher safe utensils to save time and ensure cleanliness.

- **Wooden spoons.** Choose ones with comfortable handles.

Nice-to-Have Supplies

- **Dishware (durable and chip-resistant).** From table to storage, durable, chip-resistant dishware is an ideal choice for families with young school-aged children. Choosing a pattern with a solid color allows you to dress it up with cheerful napkins.

- **Canisters.** Splurge on a brand with an air-lock feature for longer shelf-life of grains and other items.

- **Food clips.** Consider using file clips, which are typically a less expensive option.

- **Pot holders.** Consider buying a few to keep handy or oven gloves for added protection.

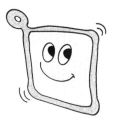

- **Vegetable brush.** Choose a sturdy model that's easy to grip firmly.

- **Plastic storage bags.** Plastic freezer bags allow removal of air and ease of labeling.

- **Permanent marker.** Keep a permanent marker in a kitchen drawer for handy labeling of plastic bags with leftovers.

Recommended Daily Intake: Calories

The recommended daily calorie intake for your child depends on many factors such as activity level, age, sex, height and weight. Counting calories is generally unnecessary, but knowing a ballpark number can help you plan a healthy diet. The chart below provides an estimate of the recommended daily calorie intake for girls and boys, age 4 to 13 years.

Recommended Daily Calorie Intake for Children			
	Sedentary*	Moderately Active**	Active***
Girls			
4 to 8 years old	1,200 to 1,400	1,400 to 1,600	1,400 to 1,800
9 to 13 years	1,400 to 1,600	1,600 to 2,000	1,800 to 2,200
Boys			
4 to 8 years old	1,200 to 1,400	1,400 to 1,600	1,600 to 2,000
9 to 13 years	1,600 to 2,000	1,800 to 2,200	2,000 to 2,600

*Less than 30 minutes of moderate physical activity per day beyond normal daily activities.
**Between 30 to 60 minutes of moderate physical activity per day beyond normal daily activities.
***More than 60 minutes of moderate physical activity per day beyond normal daily activities.
Source: Dietary Guidelines for Americans (2020-2025).

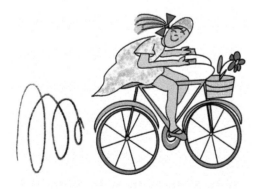

Recommended Daily "Empty Calorie" Limit

No food is forbidden, but every one counts. The chart below provides a recommended limit for "empty calorie" foods for girls and boys, age 4 to 13 years. These foods are typically high in added fat or sugar, but devoid of any nutritional value. Nonetheless, these foods won't derail an otherwise healthy diet when they make up no more than 15% of the total daily calorie intake.

Recommended "Empty Calorie" Limit (No More Than) for Girls and Boys			
	Sedentary*	**Moderately Active****	**Active****
Girls			
4 to 8 years old	180 to 210	210 to 240	210 to 270
9 to 13 years	210 to 240	240 to 300	270 to 330
Boys			
4 to 8 years old	180 to 210	210 to 240	240 to 300
9 to 13 years	240 to 300	270 to 330	300 to 390

*Less than 30 minutes of moderate physical activity per day beyond normal daily activities.
**Between 30 to 60 minutes of moderate physical activity per day beyond normal daily activities.
***More than 60 minutes of moderate physical activity per day beyond normal daily activities.
Source: Dietary Guidelines for Americans (2020-2025).

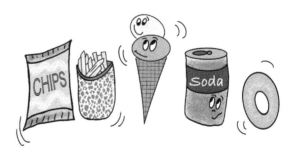

Sample Serving Sizes for Each Food Group

Fruit

One serving equals:
- 1 cup fruit
- ½ cup dried fruit
- 1 cup fruit juice*

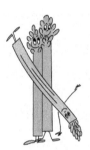

Protein and Legumes

One serving equals:
- 1 ounce meat, poultry or fish
- ¼ cup cooked dry beans
- 1 egg
- ½ ounce nuts

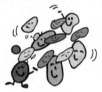

Vegetables

One serving equals:
- 1 cup raw or cooked
- 2 cups leafy greens
- 1 cup veggie juice*

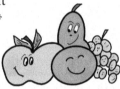

Grains

One serving equals:
- ½ cup cooked cereal, rice or pasta
- 1 slice bread
- 1 cup dry cereal
- ½ muffin
- 1 mini bagel

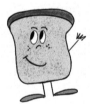

Dairy

One serving equals:
- 1 cup milk
- 1 cup yogurt
- 1½ ounce cheese

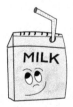

Fat

One serving equals:
- 1 teaspoon oil
- 1 teaspoon butter (1 pat)

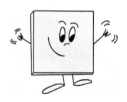

*Lower fiber option to choose less often.
Adapted from: USDA MyPlate (www.myplate.gov).

Recommended Daily Intake: Food Groups

The recommended daily food intake for your child is listed below by food group. You'll want to know how closely your child's intake matches the recommended intake for their age. To spot check, keep a one-day food record. Here's how: Tomorrow, write down all the foods and beverages your child eats, including the amounts. Remember to ask about foods eaten while at school and away from home. Compare the one-day food record to the recommended intakes listed in the table below.

Recommended Daily Servings by Food Group for Children*			
	4 to 8 years old	**9 to 13 years old**	
Food Group	**Girls and Boys**	**Girls**	**Boys**
Vegetables	1½ to 2	2 to 2½	2 to 3
Fruit	1½	1½ to 2	1½ to 2
Grains**	5	5 to 6	6 to 7
Protein, Legumes, Nuts and Seeds	4 to 5	5 to 5½	5
Dairy	2½	3	3
Oils	~3½ to 4½	~4½ to 5½	~5 to 6

* For moderately active children who get between 30 to 60 minutes of moderate physical activity per day beyond normal daily activities. Children who are more or less physically active may require more or less, respectively, to meet their calorie needs.
**At least 50% as unrefined, whole grains.
Source: Dietary Guidelines for Americans (2020-2025).

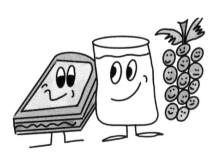

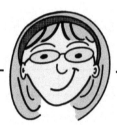

Did You Know?

Fruits and vegetables are a treasure trove of nutrients and beneficial phytochemicals that deliver powerful antioxidant protection. It's one of the reasons the Dietary Guidelines for Americans (2020-2025) recommends moderately active children, age 4 to 8 years, should consume 3 to 3½ servings of fruits and vegetables in a variety of colors every day, while older children, age 9 to 13 years, should aim for a daily intake of 3½ to 5 servings.[4]

Recommended Daily Intake: Vitamins

Vitamins: Recommended Daily Intake for Children[4,5,6,7,8,9]		
Vitamin	**4 to 8 years old**	**9 to 13 years old**
Vitamin A	400 micrograms	600 micrograms
Vitamin C	25 milligrams	45 milligrams
Vitamin D	15 micrograms (600 IU)	15 micrograms (600 IU)
Vitamin E	7 milligrams	11 milligrams
Vitamin K	55 micrograms	60 micrograms
Thiamin (Vitamin B1)	0.6 milligrams	0.9 milligrams
Riboflavin (Vitamin B2)	0.6 milligrams	0.9 milligrams
Niacin	8 milligrams	12 milligrams
Vitamin B6	0.6 milligrams	1 milligram
Folate*	200 micrograms	300 micrograms
Vitamin B12	1.2 micrograms	1.8 micrograms
Pantothenic Acid	3 milligrams	4 milligrams
Biotin	12 micrograms	20 micrograms
Choline	250 milligrams	375 milligrams
*Also known as folic acid.		

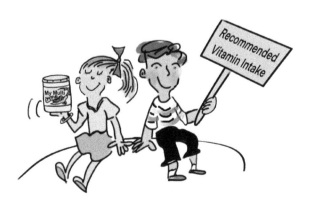

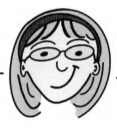

Did You Know?

Variety in your child's diet is important to help ensure an adequate amount of all the essential nutrients—over 35 vitamins, minerals and macronutrients—as well as emerging nutrients such as health-promoting phytochemicals. One of the easiest ways to boost variety is to tap into your child's quest for flavorful foods. The bonus: Trying new food taste sensations can be a fun adventure.

Recommended Daily Intake: Minerals

Minerals: Recommended Daily Intake for Children[5,6,7,8,10,11]		
Mineral	**4 to 8 years old**	**9 to 13 years old**
Calcium	1,000 milligrams	1,300 milligrams
Chromium	15 micrograms	21 micrograms (girls) 25 micrograms (boys)
Copper	440 micrograms	700 micrograms
Fluoride	1 milligram	2 milligrams
Iodine	90 micrograms	120 micrograms
Iron	10 milligrams	8 milligrams
Magnesium	130 milligrams	240 milligrams
Manganese	1.5 milligrams	1.6 milligrams (girls) 1.9 milligrams (boys)
Molybdenum	22 micrograms	34 micrograms
Phosphorus	500 milligrams	1250 milligrams
Selenium	30 micrograms	40 micrograms
Zinc	5 milligrams	8 milligrams
Potassium	2,300 milligrams	2,300 milligrams (girls)
		2,500 milligrams (boys)
Sodium	1,500 milligrams	1,800 milligrams
Chloride	1.9 grams	2.3 grams

Recommended Daily Intake: Macronutrients

Macronutrient Range: Recommended Daily Intake for Children		
Macronutrient	**4 to 8 years old**	**9 to 13 years old**
Carbohydrates	45% to 65%	45% to 65%
Protein	10% to 30%	10% to 30%
Fat	25% to 35%	25% to 35%
Linoleic Acid (Omega-6 Fat)	10 grams	10 grams (girls) 12 grams (boys)
Linolenic Acid (Omega-3 Fat)	0.9 grams	1.0 gram (girls) 1.2 grams (boys)
Fiber (per 1,000 calories)	14 grams	14 grams
Source: Dietary Guidelines for Americans (2020-2025).		

Example: A 2,000-calorie menu plan provides the following macronutrient distribution:*

Carbohydrates: 900 to 1,300 calories (225 to 325 grams)
Protein: 200 to 600 calories (50 to 150 grams)
Fat: 500 to 700 calories (56 to 78 grams)
Fiber: 28 grams

* Carbohydrates and protein contain 4 calories per gram; fat contains 9 calories per gram.

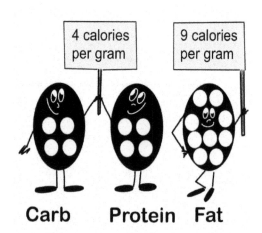

Recommended Daily Intake: Water

Every system in your child's body requires water. An adequate intake is essential to aid digestion, bring nutrients and oxygen to the cells, remove waste products and maintain normal metabolism. Foods contribute some water to your child's total daily intake, but most of it comes from drinking water and other beverages. So, encourage your child to drink up.

Water: Recommended Daily Intake for Children			
	Total Water	**From Beverages**	**From Food**
Girls			
4 to 8 years old	7 cups	5 cups	2 cups
9 to 13 years old	9 cups	7 cups	2 cups
Boys			
4 to 8 years old	7 cups	5 cups	2 cups
9 to 13 years old	10 cups	8 cups	2 cups
Institute of Medicine. *Dietary Reference Intakes for Water, Potassium, Sodium, Chloride, and Sulfate*. National Academies Press; 2005.			

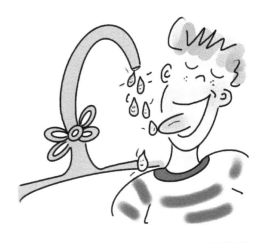

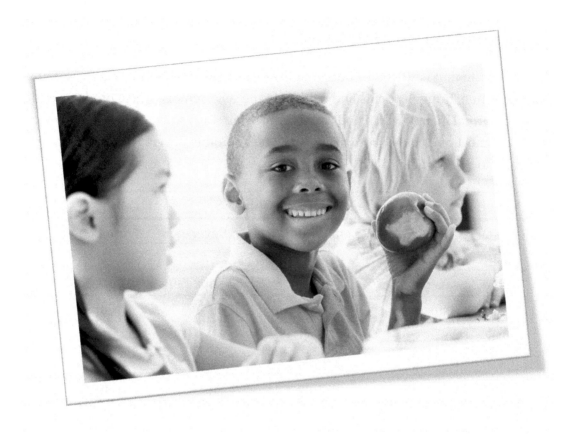

Children are like wet cement.
Whatever falls on them makes an impression.
– Dr. Haim Ginott

Glossary

Acetylcholine – An important chemical messenger in the brain for cell-to-cell communication involved in learning, memory and other functions.

Alpha-linolenic acid (ALA) – An essential omega-3 fatty acid.

Amino acid - A protein building block.

Anthocyanins – Red, purple and blue plant pigments with strong antioxidant properties.

Antioxidants – Protective nutrients such as vitamins C and E and numerous naturally occurring plant compounds. In the body, antioxidants help protect against harmful free radicals.

Biotin – A B vitamin involved in the metabolism of carbohydrates and the synthesis of fats and proteins.

Body mass index (BMI) – An estimate of body fat and predictor of overall health.

Brain-derived neurotropic factor (BDNF) – A chemical in the brain that's responsible for the development of new brain tissue.

Caffeine – A compound found in foods, beverages and over-the-counter drugs designed to fight fatigue. It has a stimulating effect that can last for several hours and a diuretic effect (increases the body's ability to expel water) that can lead to dehydration.

Calcium – A mineral essential for the formation of strong bones and teeth. It also stimulates blood clotting after injury and is required for normal muscle and nerve activity. Adequate calcium intake may reduce the risk of osteoporosis later in life.

Calorie – A unit of measure used to express the energy in foods.

Carbohydrates – The main source of energy in the diet (providing 4 calories per gram). The two main types are simple carbohydrates (simple sugars) and complex carbohydrates (starch and fiber).

Carotenoids – Plant pigments with antioxidant properties such as alpha-carotene, beta-carotene, beta-cryptoxanthin, lutein, zeaxanthin and lycopene.

Choline – A chemical cousin to the B vitamin family; serves as a building block for phosphatidylcholine.

Chromium – A trace mineral that's essential for the normal metabolism of glucose. It also influences carbohydrate, fat and protein metabolism. Refining food leads to appreciable losses of chromium.

Complex carbohydrate – A compound containing long chains of simple sugars that provides a sustained increase in energy.

Copper – A trace mineral involved in iron metabolism, nervous system functioning, bone health and the synthesis of proteins. It's an essential component of an antioxidant enzyme and also plays a role in the pigmentation of skin, hair and eyes.

Docosahexaenoic acid (DHA) – An essential omega-3 fatty acid.

Eicosapentaenoic acid (EPA) – An essential omega-3 fatty acid.

Empty calories – Foods that lack any nutritional value beyond providing calories.

Enzyme – A compound produced by cells to help activate or speed up biochemical reactions.

Fat – An essential nutrient that provides concentrated energy (9 calories per gram), contributes to the taste of food, acts as a carrier of fat-soluble vitamins and supplies essential fatty acids.

Fiber – A type of complex carbohydrate that exhibits various degrees of resistance to human digestion. It's found only in foods of plant origin.

Folic acid – Also known as folate, this B vitamin works hand in hand with vitamin B12. It's essential to regulate and maintain overall cellular health, healthy cell division and the formation of new cells, including red blood cells.

Food neophobia – A fear of new foods.

Free radicals – Unstable and highly reactive compounds that form during normal metabolism. Their production dramatically increases with exposure to sun, air pollution, smoking and other damaging environmental factors as well as from intense exercise. With an adequate intake of antioxidants, the body can neutralize free radicals before they can harm cells and tissues.

Glycemic Index (GI) – A system of ranking foods based on how they affect the rise in blood glucose (blood sugar) immediately after being consumed.

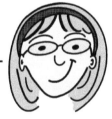

Did You Know?

One way to determine if your child is consuming enough fiber is to check stool consistency. In practical terms, simply have your child look at his or her poop in the toilet bowl before flushing. If it's a floater, it's a good indication of an adequate fiber intake. If it's a sinker, it's a sign that your child needs to eat more fiber-rich foods.

Glycogen – The main storage form of carbohydrates in the body.

Indoles – A group of phytonutrients found in broccoli, cauliflower, cabbage and other cruciferous vegetables that help activate enzymes in the body.

Iodine – As part of thyroid hormones, this mineral helps regulate growth, development and energy metabolism. Seafood, such as shellfish, fish and seaweed, are the best sources of iodine.

Iron – A trace mineral that's an essential part of hemoglobin, a compound which carries oxygen in the blood. Iron is also involved in energy metabolism. Iron deficiency anemia is a common health problem in children.

Lutein – A natural occurring carotenoid found in fruits and veggies with antioxidant properties, and one of only two carotenoids taken up by the eye to support healthy vision (the other is zeaxanthin).

Lycopene – A carotenoid that gives fruits and veggies their red and pink colors. Lycopene has been shown to provide antioxidant activity, and a diet rich in lycopene has been associated with prostate and heart health.

Macronutrient – A nutrient required in large amounts (grams) such as carbohydrate, fat, protein, fiber and water.

Magnesium – A mineral required for the normal activity of nerves and muscles (including heart muscle). It plays a role in the metabolism of ATP (cellular energy compound) and DNA (genetic material).

Manganese – A trace mineral that's necessary for the normal development of skeletal and connective tissues. It plays a role in fatty acid synthesis and carbohydrate metabolism. Low intakes of manganese may lead to porous bone.

Memory consolidation – A type of cognitive process that converts new information into a lasting memory.

Micronutrient – A nutrient, including vitamins and some minerals, that's required by the body in small amounts (milligrams or micrograms).

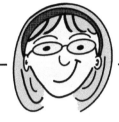

Did You Know?

An optimal intake of magnesium is linked to the ability to handle mental stress that can make kids (and adults) moody, irritable and downright grumpy. Magnesium is available in a wide variety of foods, but the richest sources are plant foods, including dark green vegetables, seeds, nuts, legumes and whole grains. Other food sources include fish and milk.[1]

Mineral – An indestructible element that cannot be broken down by heat, acid or air. Unlike a vitamin, a mineral is not produced by a living organism. A mineral that's required for human health is known as an "essential mineral."

Molybdenum – A trace mineral that's an essential part of several enzymes in the body. It may be involved in the metabolism of the hormone glucocorticoid.

Neurotoxin – A substance that causes damage to nerves or nerve tissue.

Neurotransmitter – A signaling molecule released from a nerve cell that allows it to communicate with another nerve cell, muscle, organ or other tissue.

Nerve growth factors – A naturally occurring molecule in the body that stimulates the growth and differentiation of certain sensory nerves and nerves responsible for heart rate and other automatic functions (sympathetic nerves).

Niacin (Vitamin B3) – A B vitamin that's essential for the release of energy from carbohydrates, fats and proteins. It helps maintain healthy skin and plays a role in blood glucose (blood sugar) control.

Norepinephrine – An important neurotransmitter that helps sustain attention and the ability to concentrate.

Omega-3-fatty acids – A class of fatty acids that includes DHA, the essential fatty acid that supports optimal health, especially heart, brain and eye health. An adequate dietary intake of fatty acids in this class helps counterbalance a high dietary intake of omega-6 fatty acids.

Organic foods – Chemically, a carbon-containing molecule. For foods, the U.S. Department of Agriculture (USDA) permits the use of the term on foods that meet certain standards. Organic plant foods must be grown without the use of synthetic pesticides, fungicides or inorganic fertilizers. Organic animal foods must be from animals raised on organic feed that's free of any slaughtered animal parts, allowed outside and not given antibiotics or growth hormones.

Oxidative stress – A condition that occurs when the production of free radicals exceeds the body's normal ability to neutralize and eliminate them. This condition may occur with excessive exposure to sun, air pollution, smoking and other damaging environmental factors as well as from intense exercise.

Pantothenic acid (Vitamin B5) – A B vitamin that helps release energy from foods and is a key component of fat metabolism. A significant loss of this vitamin occurs when food is processed.

Phosphatidylcholine – Also known as lecithin; a fat-like compound important for the structural integrity of cell membranes and cell-to-cell communication.

Phosphorus – An essential mineral that plays a role in the formation of bones and teeth and regulates energy release from foods. It's a component of the body's major cellular energy source, ATP, and the genetic material, DNA.

Phytonutrients – Naturally occurring plant compounds, many of which have health-protecting properties.

Protein – An organic compound made up of amino acids. Proteins are needed for growth, maintenance and repair of tissue. They are vital for the regulation of body processes, and are especially important during periods of growth. Protein provides 4 calories per gram.

Quercetin – An antioxidant in the flavonoid family that occurs naturally in foods such as apples, red grapes and tea.

Saturated fat – A type of fat that's generally solid at room temperature and commonly found in meats and foods of animal origin.

Sedentary child– A child who gets less than 30 minutes of moderate physical activity on most days.

Selenium – An essential trace mineral that acts as an antioxidant. Recent discoveries indicate selenium is also important in the metabolism of thyroid hormones.

Serotonin – An important neurotransmitter that helps sustain attention and the ability to concentrate.

Simple carbohydrate – A compound containing only one or two simple sugars that provides quick energy.

Starch – A type of complex carbohydrate consisting of long chains of simple sugars that's digestible by humans. It's found only in foods of plant origin.

Unsaturated fat – A type of fat that's generally fluid at room temperature (e.g., cooking oil) and generally derived from plants.

Vitamin – A compound, essential for life, that's produced by living organisms. Vitamins are free of calories and required by the body in only small (milligram or microgram) amounts.

Vitamin A – An essential vitamin required for vision, growth and bone development. It plays a role in the proper functioning of most organs in the body and the body's natural immune defense, including helping to maintain healthy skin and mucous membranes.

Vitamin B1 (Thiamin) – A B vitamin that assists in carbohydrate metabolism and energy production. It's required for normal nerve function and may play a role in brain function.

Vitamin B2 (Riboflavin) – A B vitamin that assists in production of energy from foods and the formation of red blood cells. It's involved in numerous metabolic reactions.

Vitamin B6 (Pyridoxine) – A B vitamin that's essential for protein metabolism, nervous system and immune system function. It also plays a role in the synthesis of hormones and red blood cells.

Vitamin B12 (Cobalamin) – A B vitamin that's essential for normal growth and the production of red blood cells. It's important for folate, carbohydrate, fat and some protein metabolism and helps maintain a healthy nervous system. Vitamin B12 is also essential for synthesis of the genetic material, DNA.

Vitamin C – A vitamin that's essential for the formation of connective tissue, bones and teeth. It's important for wound healing and gum tissue health and assists in fat breakdown (fat metabolism). Vitamin C also promotes iron absorption and provides antioxidant properties.

Vitamin D – An essential vitamin that promotes normal bone and tooth formation. It stimulates calcium and phosphorous absorption and is essential for their metabolism. Scientists believe that vitamin D has other functions unrelated to calcium. A variety of cells not involved with calcium metabolism, including certain immune cells, utilize vitamin D for purposes that are not yet understood.

Vitamin E – An essential vitamin that works as an antioxidant to protect cells, vitamin A and unsaturated fatty acids. It also plays a role in maintaining healthy red blood cells.

Vitamin K – An essential vitamin that helps synthesize proteins involved in normal blood clotting. It's also needed for the synthesis of a key protein in bone formation and may play a role in reducing hip fractures.

Water – An essential nutrient for life. It helps eliminate toxic materials in the body, transports nutrients in the body and body fluids and dissipates excess heat through perspiration.

Zinc – A trace mineral that's essential for proper growth and development and is involved in protein synthesis and digestion, wound healing, bone health and the synthesis of genetic material, DNA. It also modulates immune function and is a key component in a major antioxidant enzyme in the body.

Zeaxanthin – A natural occurring carotenoid found in fruits and veggies with antioxidant properties, and one of only two carotenoids taken up by the eye to support healthy vision (the other is lutein).

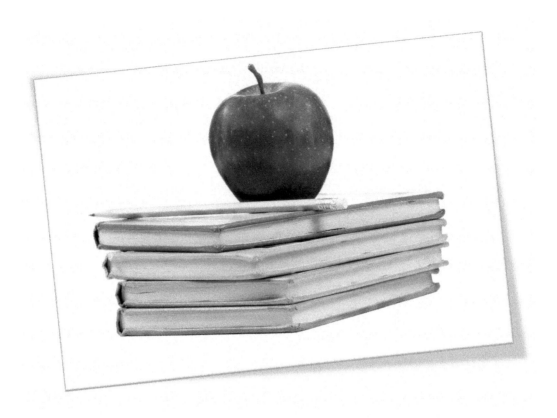

Invest a few moments in thinking.
It will pay good dividends.
— Anonymous

References

Chapter 2: September – Family Meals

1. Harrison ME, Norris ML, Obeid N, Fu M, Weinstangel H, Sampson M. Systematic review of the effects of family meal frequency on psychosocial outcomes in youth. *Can Fam Physician.* 2015;61(2):e96-106.

2. Dunford EK, Popkin BM, Ng SW. Recent trends in junk food intake in U.S. children and adolescents, 2003-2016. *Am J Prev Med.* 2020;59(1):49-58.

3. Radesky J, Chassiakos YLR, Ameenuddin N, Navsaria D; Council on Communication and Media. Digital advertising to children. *Pediatrics.* 2020;146(1):e20201681.

4. Norman J, Kelly B, McMahon AT, Boyland E, Chapman K, King L. Remember me? exposure to unfamiliar food brands in television advertising and online advergames drives children's brand recognition, attitudes, and desire to eat foods: a secondary analysis from a crossover experimental-control study with randomization at the group level. *J Acad Nutr Diet.* 2020;120(1):120-129.

5. Reid Chassiakos YL, Radesky J, Christakis D, Moreno MA, Cross C. Council on Communications and Media. Children and adolescents and digital media. *Pediatrics.* 2016;138(5).

Chapter 3: October – Feeding the Growing Brain

1. Lundqvist M, Vogel NE, Levin LÅ. Effects of eating breakfast on children and adolescents: A systematic review of potentially relevant outcomes in economic evaluations. *Food Nutr Res.* 2019;63:10.29219/fnr.v63.1618.

2. Liberali R, Kupek E, Assis MAA. Dietary patterns and childhood obesity risk: a systematic review. *Child Obes.* 2020;16(2):70-85.

3. Institute of Medicine. Food and Nutrition Board. *Dietary Reference Intakes: Thiamin, Riboflavin, Niacin, Vitamin B6, Folate, Vitamin B12, Pantothenic Acid, Biotin, and Choline.* National Academy Press; 1998.

4. von Schacky C. Importance of EPA and DHA blood levels in brain structure and function. *Nutrients.* 2021;13(4):1074.

5. Burns-Whitmore B, Froyen E, Heskey C, Parker T, San Pablo G. Alpha-linolenic and linoleic fatty acids in the vegan diet: do they require dietary reference intake/adequate intake special consideration?. *Nutrients.* 2019;11(10):2365.

6. Park Y. Dietary reference intake of n-3 polyunsaturated fatty acids for Koreans. *Nutr Res Pract.* 2022;16(suppl 1):S47-S56.

7. Sheppard KW, Cheatham CL. Omega-6/omega-3 fatty acid intake of children and older adults in the U.S.: dietary intake in comparison to current dietary recommendations and the Healthy Eating Index. *Lipids Health Dis.* 2018;17(1):43.

8. Long AC, Kuchan M, Mackey AD. Lutein as an ingredient in pediatric nutritionals. *J AOAC Int.* 2019;102(4):1034-1043.

9. Stringham JM, Johnson EJ, Hammond BR. Lutein across the lifespan: from childhood cognitive performance to the aging eye and brain. *Curr Dev Nutr.* 2019;3(7):nzz066.

10. Ma L, Liu R, Du JH, Liu T, Wu SS, Liu XH. Lutein, zeaxanthin and meso-zeaxanthin supplementation associated with macular pigment optical density. *Nutrients.* 2016;8(7):426.

11. Walk AM, Khan NA, Barnett SM, et al. From neuro-pigments to neural efficiency: the relationship between retinal carotenoids and behavioral and neuroelectric indices of cognitive control in childhood. *Int J Psychophysiol.* 2017;118:1-8.

12. Barnett SM, Khan NA, Walk AM, et al. Macular pigment optical density is positively associated with academic performance among preadolescent children. *Nutr Neurosci.* 2018;21(9):632-640.

13. Toribio-Mateas M. Harnessing the power of microbiome assessment tools as part of neuroprotective nutrition and lifestyle medicine interventions. *Microorganisms.* 2018;6(2).

14. Rowland I, Gibson G, Heinken A, et al. Gut microbiota functions: metabolism of nutrients and other food components. *Eur J Nutr.* 2018;57(1):1-24.

15. Carlson JL, Erickson JM, Lloyd BB, Slavin JL. Health effects and sources of prebiotic dietary fiber. *Curr Dev Nutr.* 2018;2(3):nzy005.

16. Sabater-Molina M, Larqué E, Torrella F, Zamora S. Dietary fructooligosaccharides and potential benefits on health. *J Physiol Biochem.* 2009;65(3):315-28.

17. Sugizaki CSA, Naves MMV. Potential prebiotic properties of nuts and edible seeds and their relationship to obesity. *Nutrients.* 2018;10(11).

Chapter 4: November – Eat Your Colors

1. Yang L, Wen KS, Ruan X, Zhao YX, Wei F, Wang Q. Response of plant secondary metabolites to environmental factors. *Molecules*. 2018;23(4):762.

2. Erb M, Kliebenstein DJ. Plant secondary metabolites as defenses, regulators, and primary metabolites: the blurred functional trichotomy. *Plant Physiol*. 2020;184(1):39-52.

3. Travica N, D'Cunha NM, Naumovski N, et al. The effect of blueberry interventions on cognitive performance and mood: a systematic review of randomized controlled trials. *Brain Behav Immun*. 2020;85:96-105.

4. Khan UM, Sevindik M, Zarrabi A, et al. Lycopene: food sources, biological activities, and human health benefits. *Oxid Med Cell Longev*. 2021:2713511.

5. USDA FoodData Central. https://fdc.nal.usda.gov

6. Mohammed HA, Khan RA. Anthocyanins: traditional uses, structural and functional variations, approaches to increase yields and products' quality, hepatoprotection, liver longevity, and commercial products. *Int J Mol Sci*. 2022;23(4):2149.

7. Haytowitz, D.B., Wu, X., Bhagwat, S. 2018. USDA Database for the Flavonoid Content of Selected Foods, Release 3.3. U.S. Department of Agriculture, Agricultural Research Service. Nutrient Data Laboratory. http://www.ars.usda.gov/nutrientdata/flav/

8. Yu J, Gleize B, Zhang L, Caris-Veyrat C, Renard CMGC. Heating tomato puree in the presence of lipids and onion: the impact of onion on lycopene isomerization. *Food Chem*. 2019;296:9-16.

9. Abdel-Aal el-SM, Akhtar H, Zaheer K, Ali R. Dietary sources of lutein and zeaxanthin carotenoids and their role in eye health. *Nutrients*. 2013;5(4):1169-1185.

10. Sharma S, Katoch V, Kumar S, Chatterjee S. Functional relationship of vegetable colors and bioactive compounds: implications in human health. *J Nutr Biochem*. 2021;92:108615.

11. U.S. Department of Agriculture and U.S. Department of Health and Human Services. Dietary Guidelines for Americans, 2020-2025. 9th ed. December 2020. https://www.dietaryguidelines.gov

12. Lu C, Toepel K, Irish R, Fenske RA, Barr DB, Bravo R. Organic diets significantly lower children's dietary exposure to organophosphorus pesticides. *Environ Health Perspect*. 2006;114(2):260-263.

13. Bradman A, Quirós-Alcalá L, Castorina R, et al. Effect of organic diet intervention on pesticide exposures in young children living in low-income urban and agricultural communities. *Environ Health Perspect.* 2015;123(10):1086-1093.

14. Hyland C, Bradman A, Gerona R, et al. Organic diet intervention significantly reduces urinary pesticide levels in U.S. children and adults. *Environ Res.* 2019;171:568-575. doi:10.1016/j.envres.2019.01.024

15. Environmental Working Group. Shoppers Guide to Pesticides in Produce™; 2023. https://www.ewg.org/foodnews/

Chapter 5: December – Sleep, De-Stress & Learn

1. Gomez AG, Genzel L. Sleep and academic performance: considering amount, quality and timing. *Curr Opin Behav Sci.* 2020;33:65-71.

2. Trosman I, Ivanenko A. Classification and epidemiology of sleep disorders in children and adolescents. *Child Adolesc Psychiatr Clin N Am.* 2021;30(1):47-64.

3. Rey AE, Guignard-Perret A, Imler-Weber F, Garcia-Larrea L, Mazza S. Improving sleep, cognitive functioning and academic performance with sleep education at school in children. *Learning and Instruction.* 2020;65:101270.

4. van Woudenberg TJ, Bevelander KE, Burk WJ, Buijzen M. The reciprocal effects of physical activity and happiness in adolescents. *Int J Behav Nutr Phys Act.* 2020;17(1):147.

5. U.S. Department of Health and Human Services. Physical Activity Guidelines for Americans, 2nd ed. US Department of Health and Human Services; 2018.

6. Terry PC, Karageorghis CI, Curran ML, Martin OV, Parsons-Smith RL. Effects of music in exercise and sport: a meta-analytic review. *Psychol Bull.* 2020;146(2):91-117.

Chapter 6: January – Pack a Power Lunch

1. Khan NA, Raine LB, Drollette ES, Scudder MR, Hillman CH. The relation of saturated fats and dietary cholesterol to childhood cognitive flexibility. *Appetite.* 2015;93:51-6.

Chapter 7: February – Kids in the Kitchen

1. Patel MD, Donovan SM, Lee SY. Considering nature and nurture in the etiology and prevention of picky eating: a narrative review. *Nutrients.* 2020;12(11):3409.

Chapter 8: March – Fit Body, Fit Brain

1. McKenna MC, Dienel GA, Sonnewald U, Waagepetersen HS, Schousbo A. Chapter 11: Energy Metabolism of the Brain. In: BradyST, Siegel GJ, Albers RW, Price DL, eds. *Basic Neurochemistry: Principles of Molecular, Cellular and Medical Neurobiology.* 8th ed. Academic Press; 2012:200-231.

2. US Department of Health and Human Services. Physical Activity Guidelines for Americans. 2nd ed. US Department of Health and Human Services; 2018.

3. Comeras-Chueca C, Marin-Puyalto J, Matute-Llorente A, Vicente-Rodriguez G, Casajus JA, Gonzalez-Aguero A. The effects of active video games on health-related physical fitness and motor competence in children and adolescents with healthy weight: a systematic review and meta-analysis. *Int J Environ Res Public Health.* 2021;18(13):6965.

4. de Greeff JW, Bosker RJ, Oosterlaan J, Visscher C, Hartman E. Effects of physical activity on executive functions, attention and academic performance in preadolescent children: a meta-analysis. *J Sci Med Sport.* 2018;21(5):501-507.

5. Karpinski C, ed. *Sports Nutrition Manual: A Handbook for Professionals.* 6th ed. Academy of Nutrition and Dietetics; 2017;112.

6. Thomas DT, Erdman KA, Burke LM. Position of the Academy of Nutrition and Dietetics, Dietitians of Canada, and the American College of Sports Medicine: nutrition and athletic performance. *J Acad Nutr Diet.* 2016;116(3):501-528.

7. Muralidharan AR, Lança C, Biswas S, et al. Light and myopia: from epidemiological studies to neurobiological mechanisms. *Ther Adv Ophthalmol.* 2021;13:1-45.

8. Gill N, Gjelsvik A, Mercurio LY, Amanullah S. Childhood obesity is associated with poor academic skills and coping mechanisms. *J Pediatr.* 2021;228:278-284.

9. CDC National Center for Health Statistics website. Prevalence of Overweight, Obesity, and Severe Obesity Among Children and Adolescents Aged 2–19 Years: United States, 1963–1965 Through 2017–2018. https://www.cdc.gov/nchs/data/hestat/obesity-child-17-18/obesity-child.htm

10. Eck KM, Delaney CL, Leary MP, et al. "My tummy tells me" cognitions, barriers and supports of parents and school-age children for appropriate portion sizes. *Nutrients.* 2018;10(8):1040.

11. Chye S, Valappil AC, Wright DJ, et al. The effects of combined action observation and motor imagery on corticospinal excitability and movement outcomes: two meta-analyses. *Neurosci Biobehav Rev.* 2022;143:104911.

12. Lindsay R, Spittle M, Larkin P. The effect of mental imagery on skill performance in sport: a systematic review. *J Sci Med Sport*. 2019;22(suppl 2):S92.

Chapter 9: April – Celebration beyond Cupcakes

1. Ricciuto L, Fulgoni VL 3rd, Gaine PC, Scott MO, DiFrancesco L. Sources of added sugars intake among the U.S. population: analysis by selected sociodemographic factors using the National Health and Nutrition Examination Survey 2011-18. *Front Nutr*. 2021;8:687643.

2. U.S. Department of Agriculture. FoodData Central database. https://fdc.nal.usda.gov

3. Pomeranz JL, Harris JL. Children's fruit "juice" drinks and FDA regulations: opportunities to increase transparency and support public health. *Am J Public Health*. 2020;110(6):871-880.

4. Nasseripour M, Newton JT, Warburton F, et al. A systematic review and meta-analysis of the role of sugar-free chewing gum on *Streptococcus mutans*. *BMC Oral Health*. 2021;21(1):217.

5. Fadó R, Molins A, Rojas R, Casals N. Feeding the Brain: Effect of Nutrients on Cognition, Synaptic Function, and AMPA Receptors. *Nutrients*. 2022;14(19):4137.

6. Fitch C, Keim KS; Academy of Nutrition and Dietetics. Position of the Academy of Nutrition and Dietetics: use of nutritive and nonnutritive sweeteners. *J Acad Nutr Diet*. 2012;112(5):739-758.

Chapter 10: May – New Foods for Curious Minds

1. Białek-Dratwa A, Szczepańska E, Szymańska D, Grajek M, Krupa-Kotara K, Kowalski O. Neophobia–a natural developmental stage or feeding difficulties for children? *Nutrients*. 2022;14(7):1521.

2. Nekitsing C, Blundell-Birtill P, Cockroft JE, Hetherington MM. Systematic review and meta-analysis of strategies to increase vegetable consumption in preschool children aged 2-5 years. *Appetite*. 2018;127:138-154.

Chapter 11: June – The Wonders of Water

1. Shah NJ, Abbas Z, Ridder D, Zimmermann M, Oros-Peusquens AM. A novel MRI-based quantitative water content atlas of the human brain. *Neuroimage*. 2022;252:119014.

2. Institute of Medicine. *Dietary Reference Intakes for Water, Potassium, Sodium, Chloride, and Sulfate*. National Academies Press; 2005.

3. Shinwell J, Defeyter MA. Investigation of summer learning loss in the UK-implications for holiday club provision. *Front Public Health*. 2017;5:270.

4. Markt SC, Nuttall E, Turman C, et al. Sniffing out significant "Pee values": genome wide association study of asparagus anosmia. *BMJ.* 2016;355:i6071.

5. Thomas DT, Erdman KA, Burke LM. Position of the Academy of Nutrition and Dietetics, Dietitians of Canada, and the American College of Sports Medicine: Nutrition and Athletic Performance. *J Acad Nutr Diet.* 2016;116(3):501-528.

6. Russo RG, Northridge ME, Wu B, Yi SS. Characterizing sugar-sweetened beverage consumption for us children and adolescents by race/ethnicity. *J Racial Ethn Health Disparities.* 2020;7(6):1100-1116.

7. National Geographic Website. One Bottle at a Time. https://education.nationalgeographic.org/resource/one-bottle-time/

8. EarthDay.org. Fact Sheet: Single Use Plastics. https://www.earthday.org/fact-sheet-single-use-plastics/

9. Canada.ca Website. Caffeine in Foods. https://www.canada.ca/en/health-canada/services/food-nutrition/food-safety/food-additives/caffeine-foods.html

Chapter 12: July – Label Reading Short Cuts

1. Supermarket Facts. FMI The Food Industry Association Website. Available at: https://www.fmi.org/our-research/supermarket-facts

2. Juan W, Ferguson M, Boyer M, Henderson C, Kevala J. Methodology used to modernize the reference amounts customarily consumed/serving size for the nutrition facts label. *J Food Compost Anal.* 2019;83:103297.

3. U.S. Department of Agriculture and U.S. Department of Health and Human Services. Dietary Guidelines for Americans, 2020-2025. 9th ed. December 2020. Available at: https://www.dietaryguidelines.gov.

4. Ginter E, Simko V. New data on harmful effects of trans-fatty acids. *Bratisl Lek Listy.* 2016;117(5):251-253.

5. Pipoyan D, Stepanyan S, Stepanyan S, et al. The effect of trans fatty acids on human health: regulation and consumption patterns. *Foods.* 2021;10(10):2452.

6. Oteng AB, Kersten S. Mechanisms of Action of trans Fatty Acids. *Adv Nutr.* 2020;11(3):697-708.

7. Nagpal T, Sahu JK, Khare SK, Bashir K, Jan K. Trans fatty acids in food: a review on dietary intake, health impact, regulations and alternatives. *J Food Sci.* 2021;86(12):5159-5174.

8. Amico A, Wootan MG, Jacobson MF, Leung C, Willett AW. The demise of artificial trans fat: a history of a public health achievement. *Milbank Q.* 2021;99(3):746-770.

9. Gebauer SK, Baer DJ. Trans-fatty acids: health effects, recommendations, and regulations. Ref Module Food Sci. 2022:1-5. Update of: Gebauer SK, Baer DJ. Trans-fatty acids: health effects, recommendations, and regulations. In: Caballero B, ed. *Encyclopedia of Human Nutrition.* 3rd ed. Academic Press;2013:288-292.

10. Quezada JC, Etter A, Ghazoul J, Buttler A, Guillaume T. Carbon neutral expansion of oil palm plantations in the Neotropics. *Sci Adv.* 2019;5(11):eaaw4418.

11. Brouillard AM, Deych E, Canter C, Rich MW. Trends in sodium intake in children and adolescents in the US and the impact of US Department of Agriculture guidelines: NHANES 2003-2016. *J Pediatr.* 2020;225:117-123.

12. Paglia L, Friuli S, Colombo S, Paglia M. The effect of added sugars on children's health outcomes: Obesity, Obstructive Sleep Apnea Syndrome (OSAS), Attention-Deficit/Hyperactivity Disorder (ADHD) and Chronic Diseases. *Eur J Paediatr Dent.* 2019;20(2):127-132.

Chapter 13: August – Prep for a New School Year

1. USDA MyPlate, U.S. Department of Agriculture. What is MyPlate? https://www.myplate.gov

2. Paruthi S, Brooks LJ, D'Ambrosio C, Hall WA, Kotagal S, et al. Consensus statement of the American Academy of Sleep Medicine on the recommended amount of sleep for healthy children: methodology and discussion. *J Clin Sleep Med.* 2016;12):1549-1561.

3. Back-to-school tips. American Academy of Pediatrics. https://healthychildren.org

Chapter 14: Go for the Goal

1. Vigar V, Myers S, Oliver C, Arellano J, Robinson S, Leifert C. A systematic review of organic versus conventional food consumption: is there a measurable benefit on human health?. *Nutrients.* 2019;12(1):7.

2. Bouzari A, Holstege D, Barrett DM. Vitamin retention in eight fruits and vegetables: a comparison of refrigerated and frozen storage. *J Agric Food Chem.* 2015;63(3):957-962.

3. Food and Agriculture Organization of the United Nations (FAO). Fats and fatty acids in human nutrition. Report of an expert consultation. *FAO Food Nutr Pap.* 2010;91:1-166.

4. U.S. Department of Agriculture and U.S. Department of Health and Human Services. Dietary Guidelines for Americans, 2020-2025. 9th ed. December 2020. https://www.dietaryguidelines.gov

5. Institute of Medicine. *Dietary Reference Intakes for Calcium and Vitamin D (2011); and Dietary Reference Intakes for Sodium and Potassium.* National Academies Press.

6. Institute of Medicine. *Dietary Reference Intakes for Calcium, Phosphorous, Magnesium, Vitamin D, and Fluoride.* National Academies Press; 1997.

7. Institute of Medicine. *Dietary Reference Intakes for Vitamin A, Vitamin K, Arsenic, Boron, Chromium, Copper, Iodine, Iron, Manganese, Molybdenum, Nickel, Silicon, Vanadium, and Zinc.* National Academies Press; 2001.

8. Institute of Medicine. *Dietary Reference Intakes for Vitamin C, Vitamin E, Selenium, and Carotenoids.* National Academies Press; 2000.

9. Institute of Medicine. *Dietary Reference Intakes for Thiamin, Riboflavin, Niacin, Vitamin B6, Folate, Vitamin B12, Pantothenic Acid, Biotin, and Choline.* National Academies Press; 1998.

10. U.S. Department of Agriculture and U.S. Department of Health and Human Services. Dietary Guidelines for Americans, 2020-2025. 9th ed. December 2020. https://www.dietaryguidelines.gov.

11. Institute of Medicine. *Dietary Reference Intakes for Water, Potassium, Sodium, Chloride, and Sulfate.* National Academies Press; 2005.

Glossary

1. Pickering G, Mazur A, Trousselard M, et al. Magnesium status and stress: the vicious circle concept revisited. *Nutrients.* 2020;12(12):3672.

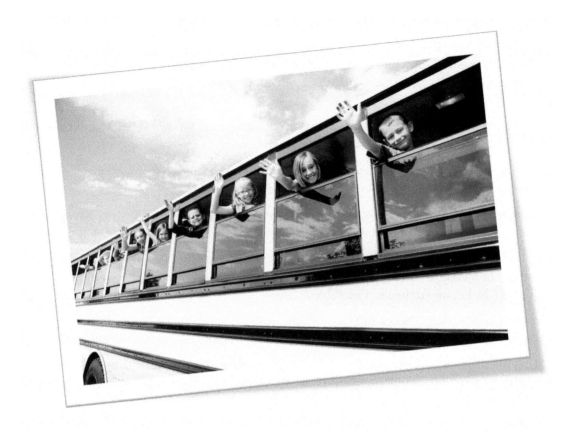

The journey is the reward.
– Chinese proverb

Index

Acknowledgements

Many thanks to our fearless copy reviewers, Brad Williams, Patti Crandall, Maureen Dunn and Ernest Noble, who provided insightful comments on drafts too numerous to count. Thank you from the bottom of our hearts. You rock!

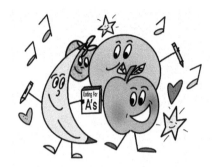

About the Authors

Kathleen Dunn, MPH, RD, and Lorna Williams, MPH, RD, are registered dietitians who have been collaborating on health and nutrition projects for over 25 years since their graduate school days (Go Bruins!). Lorna's a big fan of a "Make it Fun" approach, while Kathleen gravitates to a "Need to Know" method. It's the perfect blend of whimsy and science to deliver nutrition information that matters to you.

Kathleen and Lorna are members of the Academy of Nutrition and Dietetics. Kathleen holds a bachelor's degree in biological sciences from the University of California, Irvine, and a master's degree in public health nutrition from the University of California, Los Angeles. Lorna holds two bachelor degrees from the University of California, Berkeley, one in physiology and another in nutrition and food sciences, and a master's degree in public health nutrition from the University of California, Los Angeles.